Transfusion Medicine

Editors

JEANNE E. HENDRICKSON
CHRISTOPHER A. TORMEY

HEMATOLOGY/ONCOLOGY CLINICS OF NORTH AMERICA

www.hemonc.theclinics.com

Consulting Editors
GEORGE P. CANELLOS
H. FRANKLIN BUNN

June 2016 • Volume 30 • Number 3

ELSEVIER

1600 John F. Kennedy Boulevard • Suite 1800 • Philadelphia, Pennsylvania, 19103-2899

http://www.theclinics.com

HEMATOLOGY/ONCOLOGY CLINICS OF NORTH AMERICA Volume 30, Number 3
June 2016 ISSN 0889-8588, ISBN 13: 978-0-323-44616-7

Editor: Jennifer Flynn-Briggs
Developmental Editor: Kristen Helm

Hematology/Oncology Clinics (ISSN 0889-8588) is published bimonthly by Elsevier Inc., 360 Park Avenue South, New York, NY 10010-1710. Months of issue are February, April, June, August, October, and December. Business and Editorial Offices: 1600 John F. Kennedy Blvd., Ste. 1800, Philadelphia, PA 19103—2899. Customer Service Office: 3251 Riverport Lane, Maryland Heights, MO 63043. Periodicals postage paid at New York, NY and at additional mailing offices. Subscription prices are $385.00 per year (domestic individuals), $707.00 per year (domestic institutions), $100.00 per year (domestic students/residents), $440.00 per year (Canadian individuals), $875.00 per year (Canadian institutions) $520.00 per year (international individuals), $875.00 per year (international institutions), and $255.00 per year (international and Canadian students/residents). International air speed delivery is included in all Clinics subscription prices. All prices are subject to change without notice. **POSTMASTER:** Send address changes to Hematology/Oncology Clinics of North America, Elsevier Health Sciences Division, Subscription Customer Service, 3251 Riverport Lane, Maryland Heights, MO 63043. Customer Service (orders, claims, online, change of address): Elsevier Health Sciences Division, Subscription **Customer Service, 3251 Riverport Lane, Maryland Heights, MO 63043. Tel: 1-800-654-2452 (U.S. and Canada); 314-447-8871 (outside U.S. and Canada). Fax: 314-447-8029. E-mail: journalscustomerservice-usa@elsevier.com (for print support); journalsonlinesupport-usa@elsevier.com (for online support).**

Reprints. For copies of 100 or more, of articles in this publication, please contact the Commercial Reprints Department, Elsevier Inc., 360 Park Avenue South, New York, New York 10010-1710; Tel.: 212-633-3874, Fax: 212-633-3820, E-mail: reprints@elsevier.com.

Hematology/Oncology Clinics of North America is covered in MEDLINE/PubMed (Index Medicus), EMBASE/ Excerpta Medica, and BIOSIS.

Contributors

CONSULTING EDITORS

GEORGE P. CANELLOS, MD
William Rosenberg Professor of Medicine, Department of Medical Oncology, Dana-Farber Cancer Institute, Boston, Massachusetts

H. FRANKLIN BUNN, MD
Professor of Medicine, Division of Hematology, Brigham and Women's Hospital, Harvard Medical School, Boston, Massachusetts

EDITORS

JEANNE E. HENDRICKSON, MD
Associate Professor of Laboratory Medicine and Pediatrics, Departments of Laboratory Medicine and Pediatrics, Yale University School of Medicine, New Haven, Connecticut

CHRISTOPHER A. TORMEY, MD
Associate Professor of Laboratory Medicine, Department of Laboratory Medicine, Yale University School of Medicine, New Haven, Connecticut; Pathology and Laboratory Medicine Service, VA Connecticut Healthcare System, West Haven, Connecticut

AUTHORS

RACHEL S. BERCOVITZ, MD, MS
Associate Medical Director, Medical Sciences Institute, BloodCenter of Wisconsin; Assistant Professor of Pathology and Pediatrics, Medical College of Wisconsin, Milwaukee, Wisconsin

JEFFREY L. CARSON, MD
Provost - New Brunswick; Rutgers Biomedical and Health Sciences; Vice Chair, Research Richard C Reynolds Professor of Medicine, Rutgers Robert Wood Johnson Medical School, Rutgers, New Jersey

STELLA T. CHOU, MD
Assistant Professor, Department of Pediatrics, Abramson Research Center, The Children's Hospital of Philadelphia, Perelman School of Medicine, University of Pennsylvania, Philadelphia, Pennsylvania

GEMMA L. CRIGHTON, BHB, MBChB
Department of Epidemiology and Preventive Medicine, The Alfred Centre, Monash University, Melbourne; Australian Red Cross Blood Service, West Melbourne; The Royal Children's Hospital, Department of Haematology, Melbourne, Victoria, Australia

MELISSA M. CUSHING, MD
Associate Professor, Department of Pathology and Laboratory Medicine, Division of Transfusion Medicine and Cellular Therapy, Weill Cornell Medical College, New York, New York

DANA V. DEVINE, PhD
Professor of Pathology and Laboratory Medicine, Centre for Blood Research, University of British Columbia, Vancouver, British Columbia, Canada; Chief Medical and Scientific Officer, Canadian Blood Services, Ottawa, Ontario, Canada

NANCY M. DUNBAR, MD
Departments of Pathology and Medicine, Dartmouth-Hitchcock Medical Center, Lebanon, New Hampshire

LISE J. ESTCOURT, MB, BChir
Radcliffe Department of Medicine, National Health Service Blood and Transplant, Oxford University Hospitals NHS Trust, John Radcliffe Hospital, University of Oxford, Oxford, United Kingdom

ROSS M. FASANO, MD
Assistant Director, Transfusion, Tissue, and Apheresis, Children's Healthcare of Atlanta; Associate Director, Grady Health System Transfusion Services; Departments of Clinical Pathology and Pediatric Hematology, Emory University School of Medicine, Atlanta, Georgia

STEFANIE K. FOREST, MD, PhD
Resident, Department of Pathology and Cell Biology, Columbia University Medical Center, New York-Presbyterian Hospital, New York, New York

ERIC A. GEHRIE, MD
Department of Laboratory Medicine, Yale University School of Medicine, New Haven, Connecticut

JEANNE E. HENDRICKSON, MD
Associate Professor of Laboratory Medicine and Pediatrics, Departments of Laboratory Medicine and Pediatrics, Yale University School of Medicine, New Haven, Connecticut

ELDAD A. HOD, MD
Associate Professor, Department of Pathology and Cell Biology, Columbia University Medical Center, New York-Presbyterian Hospital, New York, New York

YEN-MICHAEL S. HSU, MD, PhD
Assistant Professor, Department of Pathology and Laboratory Medicine, Division of Transfusion Medicine and Cellular Therapy, Weill Cornell Medical College, New York, New York

CASSANDRA D. JOSEPHSON, MD
Professor of Pathology and Pediatrics, Emory University School of Medicine, Children's Healthcare of Atlanta, Atlanta, Georgia

TAHIR MEHMOOD, MD
Division of Hospital Internal Medicine, Department of Internal Medicine, Mayo Clinic, Rochester, Minnesota

NAREG ROUBINIAN, MD, MPHTM
Assistant Clinical Investigator, Blood Systems Research Institute; Assistant Adjunct
Professor, Department of Laboratory Medicine, University of California, San Francisco,
San Francisco, California

WILLIAM J. SAVAGE, MD, PhD
Associate Medical Director, Transfusion Medicine, Brigham and Women's Hospital;
Assistant Professor of Pathology, Harvard Medical School, Boston, Massachusetts

PETER SCHUBERT, PhD
Clinical Associate Professor of Pathology and Laboratory Medicine, Centre for Blood
Research, University of British Columbia; Research Associate, Canadian Blood Services,
Vancouver, British Columbia, Canada

SIMON J. STANWORTH, MD, DPhil
Radcliffe Department of Medicine, National Health Service Blood and Transplant, Oxford
University Hospitals NHS Trust, John Radcliffe Hospital, University of Oxford, Oxford,
United Kingdom

MICHELLE TAYLOR, MD
Transfuse Solutions, Inc, Byron, Minnesota

ALAN TINMOUTH, MD, MSc, FRCPC
Associate Professor, Faculty of Medicine, Department of Medicine; Department of
Pathology and Laboratory Medicine, Ottawa Hospital, University of Ottawa; Clinical
Epidemiology Program, University of Ottawa Centre for Transfusion Research, Ottawa
Health Research Institute, Ottawa, Ontario, Canada

CHRISTOPHER A. TORMEY, MD
Associate Professor of Laboratory Medicine, Department of Laboratory Medicine, Yale
University School of Medicine, New Haven, Connecticut; Pathology and Laboratory
Medicine Service, VA Connecticut Healthcare System, West Haven, Connecticut

JEFFREY L. WINTERS, MD
Division of Transfusion Medicine, Department of Laboratory Medicine and Pathology,
Mayo Clinic, Rochester, Minnesota

ERICA M. WOOD, MBBS
Assistant Professor, Department of Epidemiology and Preventive Medicine, The Alfred
Centre, Monash University; Monash Health, Department of Haematology, Victoria,
Australia

Contents

> Anemia in patients with malignancy is common as a consequence of their
> disease and treatment. Substantial progress has been made in the man-
> agement of anemia with red blood cell transfusion in acute conditions,
> such as bleeding and infection, through the performance of large clinical
> trials. These trials suggest that transfusion at lower hemoglobin thresholds
> (restrictive transfusion ~7-8 g/dL) is safe and in some cases superior to
> higher transfusion thresholds (liberal transfusion ~9-10 g/dL). However,
> additional studies are needed in patients with malignancy to understand
> best practice in relation to quality of life as well as clinical outcomes.

> Patients with hematologic malignancies frequently become thrombocyto-
> penic as a result of their underlying malignancy or treatments, including
> cytotoxic chemotherapy and hematopoietic stem cell transplantation
> and are at increased risk of hemorrhage. Prophylactic platelet transfusions
> are aimed at preventing severe or life-threatening hemorrhage. This review
> summarizes recent evidence, including the need for prophylactic platelet
> transfusions, the optimal dose, platelet transfusion triggers, and risk fac-
> tors for bleeding. It also discusses controversies surrounding platelet
> transfusions in this population.

> Frozen plasma is a commonly used blood product. The primary indications
> for frozen plasma are the treatment and prevention of bleeding in patients
> with prolonged coagulation tests. However, there is a lack of well-
> conducted clinical trials to determine the appropriate indications for frozen
> plasma. The rationale and evidence for frozen plasma transfusions are re-
> viewed, including the evidence or lack of evidence supporting common in-
> dications. Targeting indications in which frozen plasma transfusions are
> clearly not beneficial as supported by the current evidence provides an op-
> portunity to improve the current use of frozen plasma and reduce adverse
> transfusion events.

Peripheral blood stem cell collection is an effective approach to obtain a hematopoietic graft for stem cell transplantation. Developing hematopoietic stem/progenitor cell (HSPC) mobilization methods and collection algorithms have improved efficiency, clinical outcomes, and cost effectiveness. Differences in mobilization mechanisms may change the HSPC content harvested and result in different engraftment kinetics and complications. Patient-specific factors can affect mobilization. Incorporating these factors in collection algorithms and improving assays for evaluating mobilization further extend the ability to obtain sufficient HSPCs for hematopoietic repopulation. Technological advance and innovations in leukapheresis have improved collection efficiency and reduced adverse effects.

Red blood cell (RBC) transfusion therapy is a key component of comprehensive management of patients with sickle cell disease (SCD) and has increased over time as a means of primary and secondary stroke prevention. RBC transfusions also prove to be lifesaving for many acute sickle cell–related complications. Although episodic and chronic transfusion therapy has significantly improved the morbidity and mortality of patients with SCD, transfusions are not without adverse effects. This review addresses RBC transfusion methods, evidence-based and/or expert panel–based consensus on indications for chronic and episodic transfusion indications, and strategies to prevent and manage transfusion-related complications.

Pathogen inactivation technologies represent a shift in blood safety from a reactive approach to a proactive protective strategy. Commercially available technologies demonstrate effective killing of most viruses, bacteria, and parasites and are capable of inactivating passenger leukocytes in blood products. The use of pathogen inactivation causes a decrease in the parameters of products that can be readily measured in laboratory assays but that do not seem to cause any alteration in hemostatic effect of plasma or platelet transfusions. Effort needs to be made to further develop these technologies so that the negative quality impact is ameliorated without reducing the pathogen inactivation effectiveness.

Transfusion reactions are common occurrences, and clinicians who order or transfuse blood components need to be able to recognize adverse sequelae of transfusion. The differential diagnosis of any untoward clinical event should always consider adverse sequelae of transfusion, even when transfusion occurred weeks earlier. There is no pathognomonic sign or symptom that differentiates a transfusion reaction from other potential medical problems, so vigilance is required during and after transfusion when a patient presents with a change in clinical status. This review covers the presentation, mechanisms, and management of transfusion reactions that are commonly encountered, and those that can be life-threatening.

Red blood cell (RBC) transfusion is a cornerstone of the management of patients with hematology/oncology disorders. However, a potentially deleterious consequence of transfusion is the development of alloantibodies against blood group antigens present on RBCs. Such alloantibodies can be an obstacle in providing compatible units for transfusion. Providers in this arena must fully understand the testing performed by blood banks, as well as the consequences of detected antibodies. This article reviews immunohematologic tests, describes how autoimmune hemolytic anemia is classified by autoantibodies, outlines RBC alloimmunization rates, and presents strategies to prevent/mitigate the impact of RBC alloimmunization.

Blood component modifications can be performed by the hospital blood bank for select clinical indications. In general, modification of blood components increases costs and may delay availability of the blood component because of the additional time required for some modification steps. However, the benefit of blood product modification may outweigh these concerns. Common modifications include leukoreduction, irradiation, volume reduction, splitting, and washing. Modification availability and selection practice may vary from hospital to hospital. In this article, available blood component modifications are described along with the benefits, drawbacks, and specific clinical indications supporting their use.

Platelet refractoriness occurs when there is an inadequate response to platelet transfusions, which typically has nonimmune causes, but is also associated with alloantibodies to human leukocyte antigens (HLAs) and/or human platelet antigens. Immune-mediated platelet refractoriness is suggested when a 10-minute to 1-hour corrected count increment of less than $5 \times 10^9/L$ is observed after 2 sequential transfusions using ABO-identical, freshest available platelets. When these antibodies are identified, one of three strategies should be used for identifying compatible platelet units: HLA matching, crossmatching, and antibody specificity prediction. These strategies seem to offer similar results in terms of posttransfusion platelet increments.

Thrombotic microangiopathies are a heterogeneous group of inherited and acquired disorders sharing a common clinical presentation of microangiopathic hemolytic anemia, thrombocytopenia, and organ damage. These disorders have been treated with plasma exchange (TPE) based on randomized controlled trials, which found this therapy to be effective in thrombotic thrombocytopenic purpura (TTP). For the remaining disorders, low- to very low-quality evidence exists for the use of TPE. When TPE is applied, the treatment regimen used for TTP is usually applied. There is a need for further evaluation of the role of TPE in the treatment of thrombotic microangiopathies other than TTP.

Pediatric patients with malignancies or benign hematologic diseases are a heterogeneous group with complicated underlying pathophysiologies leading to their requirements for transfusion therapy. Common practice among pediatric hematologists, oncologists, and transplant physicians is to transfuse stable patients' red cells to maintain a hemoglobin greater than 7 or 8 g/dL and transfuse platelets to maintain a count greater than 10,000 or 20,000 platelets/μL. This review compiles data from myriad studies performed in pediatric patients to give readers the knowledge needed to make an informed choice when considering different management strategies for the transfusion of red blood cells, platelets, plasma, and granulocytes.

HEMATOLOGY/ONCOLOGY
CLINICS OF NORTH AMERICA

ISSUE OF RELATED INTEREST

Clinics in Perinatology, September 2015 (Vol. 42, Issue 3)
Neonatal Hematology and Transfusion Medicine
Robert D. Christensen, Sandra E. Juul, and Antonio Del Vecchio, *Editors*
Available at: http://www.perinatology.theclinics.com/

THE CLINICS ARE AVAILABLE ONLINE!
Access your subscription at:
www.theclinics.com

Preface

Transfusion Medicine

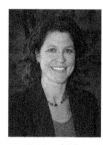 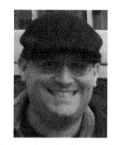

Jeanne E. Hendrickson, MD   Christopher A. Tormey, MD
Editors

Transfusion is essential for the care of a great number of individuals with Hematologic and Oncologic disorders; pediatric and adult patients alike often require red blood cell (RBC), platelet, plasma, or other blood component transfusions during their treatment courses. Because of the close relationship between Transfusion Medicine/Apheresis and Hematology/Oncology, it is imperative that clinicians in these arenas understand the advancements and challenges in each of their respective fields. Over the course of the past few decades, the investigative and clinical foci of Transfusion Services/Blood Banks has shifted from optimization of component processing/storage and reduction in infectious disease transmission for viruses such as HIV to better defining evidence-based criteria for blood component utilization, furthering our understanding of the noninfectious serious hazards of transfusion, and minimizing other transfusion-related complications. In this regard, recently completed randomized, controlled trials have changed the face of transfusion practice, resulting in the implementation of evidence-based transfusion guidelines. The recognition, prevention, and treatment of noninfectious transfusion complexities have greatly advanced as well.

Our goal in this issue of *Hematology/Oncology Clinics of North America* dedicated to Transfusion Medicine is to present practical and clinically relevant reviews on topics reflecting the current state of Immunohematology, Blood Banking, and Apheresis. Some of our chosen authors are Internists and others are Pediatricians; some are trained in Pathology/Laboratory Medicine, and others are trained in Hematology/Oncology. All are experts in Transfusion Medicine. The topics chosen include evidence-based studies of RBC, platelet, and plasma transfusion; special considerations for transfusion of pediatric or adult patients with oncologic diseases or hemoglobinopathies; management of the platelet refractory patient; approach and management of patients with microangiopathic hemolytic anemias; interpretation of immunohematologic testing; relevance of autoantibodies and alloantibodies detected in Hematology/Oncology patients; considerations of blood product modifications; adverse sequelae of transfusion; and stem cell mobilization and collection.

Hematol Oncol Clin N Am 30 (2016) xiii–xiv
http://dx.doi.org/10.1016/j.hoc.2016.02.001
0889-8588/16/$ – see front matter © 2016 Published by Elsevier Inc.

hemonc.theclinics.com

Despite continued improvements in transfusion safety, much room remains for additional optimization of transfusion management and strategies, particularly for Hematology/Oncology patients. Such optimization will require an interdisciplinary approach involving Transfusion Medicine/Apheresis and Hematology/Oncology providers alike. Areas ripe for optimization include those that further increase transfusion safety, those that conserve limited resources (taking personnel, blood product, and economic resources into consideration), and those that explore poorly understood or little studied areas of practice. This issue not only draws into focus advancements that have been made in practice but also highlights outstanding questions that remain to be answered.

As the editors of this special issue, we are extremely grateful to Dr Frank Bunn and Elsevier for their appreciation of the role of Transfusion Medicine in Hematology/Oncology practice, and for their help in making this work a reality. We would also like to express our thanks to the authors for their dedication to Transfusion Medicine, for their willingness to share their expertise, and for taking on the task of composing brief yet thorough articles with Hematology/Oncology clinicians in mind. We hope that a better understanding of current issues in Transfusion Medicine will strengthen future studies and will ultimately improve care for Hematology/Oncology patients.

Jeanne E. Hendrickson, MD
Yale University School of Medicine
Departments of Laboratory Medicine and Pediatrics
330 Cedar Street, Clinic Building 405
PO Box 208035
New Haven, CT 06520-8035, USA

Christopher A. Tormey, MD
VA Connecticut Healthcare System
Pathology and Laboratory Medicine Service
Yale University School of Medicine
Department of Laboratory Medicine
55 Park Street, Room 435B
New Haven, CT 06519, USA

E-mail addresses:
jeanne.hendrickson@yale.edu (J.E. Hendrickson)
christopher.tormey@yale.edu (C.A. Tormey)

Red Blood Cell Transfusion Strategies in Adult and Pediatric Patients with Malignancy

Nareg Roubinian, MD, MPHTM[a,b,*], Jeffrey L. Carson, MD[c]

KEYWORDS

- Randomized clinical trials • RBC transfusion • Malignancy • Bleeding

KEY POINTS

- Randomized clinical trials of red blood cell transfusion practice have provided high-quality evidence in the management of common complications of cancer.
- The preponderance of clinical trial data supports using restrictive transfusion strategies (hemoglobin levels between 7 and 8 g/dL) in most hospitalized medical and surgical patients.
- Additional studies are needed to understand best practice in the management of anemia in cancer patients with a focus on quality of life in addition to clinical outcomes.

INTRODUCTION

Anemia is common in patients with malignancy and has been associated with increased morbidity and mortality.[1] Its incidence has been correlated with advancing cancer stage and declining functional status at the time of diagnosis.[2] The severity of anemia has been found to be proportional to aberrations in inflammatory cytokines as well as hepcidin, ferritin, and erythropoietin levels.[3]

The cause of anemia in the setting of malignancy is often multifactorial and as with anemia in general includes 3 broad categories: decreased production, increased destruction, and acute blood loss. In addition to anemia related to suppression of erythropoietin, infection, and decreased red blood cell (RBC) survival owing to autoantibodies, causes specific to malignancy include direct effects of a neoplasm such

[a] Blood Systems Research Institute, 270 Masonic Avenue, San Francisco, CA 94118, USA; [b] Department of Laboratory Medicine, University of California, San Francisco, 270 Masonic Avenue, San Francisco, CA 94118, USA; [c] Research, Rutgers Robert Wood Johnson Medical School, Rutgers Biomedical and Health Sciences, Rutgers, The State University of New Jersey, 125 Paterson Street, New Brunswick, NJ 08901, USA
* Corresponding author. Blood Systems Research Institute, 270 Masonic Avenue, San Francisco, CA 94118.
E-mail address: Nareg.Roubinian@ucsf.edu

Hematol Oncol Clin N Am 30 (2016) 529–540
http://dx.doi.org/10.1016/j.hoc.2016.01.001
0889-8588/16/$ – see front matter © 2016 Elsevier Inc. All rights reserved.
hemonc.theclinics.com

as leukemic infiltration of the bone marrow as well as the effects of chemotherapy and radiation.[4]

Patients with malignancy often undergo intensive medical and surgical therapies to treat their disease. The prevalence of anemia in patients varies by the type of malignancy and the time course of diagnosis and treatment with published rates ranging from 30% to 90%.[1,5–7] Surgical treatment of malignancy often accepts significant blood loss and results in intraoperative or postoperative anemia. In parallel, medical treatment with chemotherapy often results in a hypoproliferative state and subsequent anemia. This is particularly true for patients requiring myeloablative chemotherapy or hematopoietic stem cell transplantation, who almost universally develop severe anemia that necessitates RBC transfusion.[6,8] During and after therapy, it is also not uncommon for cancer outpatients to require RBC transfusions intermittently for weeks or months.

With the performance of many randomized clinical trials there has been significant progress in understanding when to transfuse RBCs in hospitalized medical and surgical patients. Although these clinical trials were not focused on patients with malignancy, many of them included such patients and provide high-quality evidence in the management of common complications of cancer such as acute bleeding and infection.

Clinical trials to date have focused on acute conditions requiring hospitalization, and little evidence exists in the management of chronic anemia such as that of patients with hematologic malignancy. The current controversy for the use of RBCs includes the optimal hemoglobin (Hgb) trigger for transfusion and the impact of different transfusion strategies on quality of life for both inpatients and outpatients. Most outcomes collected in clinical trials relate to mortality and morbidity outcomes, such as cardiac events and hospital duration of stay. Functional status and quality of life have not been outcomes in almost all of these studies, despite oncologic society guidelines advising RBC transfusions be administered to maintain quality of life.[9,10]

In this paper, we review the randomized clinical trials evaluating RBC transfusion in the management of anemia related to common complications of malignancy. We begin by describing the goals of therapy in acute and chronic settings. We then review the risks of anemia and summarize current clinical trial data and their role in the development of society guidelines for RBC transfusion practice.

GOALS AND RISKS OF RED BLOOD CELL TRANSFUSION

The often-stated goal of RBC transfusion is to improve oxygen delivery to the tissues. However, the measurement of oxygen delivery is challenging and thresholds for transfusion are generally well above the level needed for tissue oxygenation.[11] In clinical trials, the impact of RBC transfusion has been measured in relation to symptoms and clinical events. In hospitalized patients, the goal of transfusion is to maximize survival and minimize morbid events such as infection and myocardial infarction. In contrast, the goals of RBC transfusion for chronically anemic patients with hematologic conditions or malignancies are to enhance quality of life and function while minimizing the side effects of chronic exposure to transfusion.[12] Thus, in acute settings, studies generally focus on mortality and morbidity whereas in chronic settings they focus on symptoms and function.

RBC transfusions include biologically active products that may induce immune responses and expand vascular volume. With advances in transfusion medicine, complications related to transfusion-transmitted infections, transfusion-related acute lung injury, and severe hemolytic reactions have become uncommon.[13] However, immune modulation, iron overload, or prothrombotic effects related to transfusion may have short- and long-term clinical sequelae.

The immunosuppressive activity of allogeneic blood, particularly the leukocyte component, has been known since early studies of renal allograft survival.[14,15] This phenomenon, termed transfusion-related immunomodulation, has been associated with postoperative infections, tumor recurrence, and nosocomial infections in critically ill patients. Transfusion-related immunomodulation is of particular interest in patients with malignancy who are at increased risk of infection owing to the effects of chemotherapy on mucosal barriers in addition to immune deficits related to underlying disease. Thus, RBC transfusion carries with it a spectrum of beneficial and adverse effects that vary depending on the clinical setting.

RISKS FROM ANEMIA

Symptoms and complications of anemia tend to be associated with more severe reductions in Hgb levels. According to the World Health Organization and the National Cancer Institute, normal values for Hgb are 12 to 16 g/dL in women and 14 to 18 g/dL in men, and grading of anemia is as follows: mild (grade 1), Hgb from 10 g/dL to the lower limit of normal; moderate (grade 2), Hgb 8 to 9.9 g/dL; severe (grade 3), Hgb 6.5 to 7.9 g/dL; and life threatening (grade 4), Hgb less than 6.5 g/dL.[4]

In general, moderate anemia is thought to have few associated symptoms, owing to compensatory mechanisms (increased cardiac output and 2,3 diphosphoglycerate levels, among others) that preserve oxygen transport. Historically, clinical practice was to correct moderate anemia with RBC transfusion with the goal of minimizing morbidity and mortality and treating related signs and symptoms.

Our understanding of the risks associated with anemia was advanced by study of patients undergoing surgery who refused blood transfusion.[16] An analysis of 1,958 patients of the Jehovah's Witness faith who underwent an operative procedure found that morbidity and mortality did not increase significantly until the preoperative Hgb decreased to less than 8 g/dL. As the preoperative Hgb decreased, the risk of death increased and increased significantly when either preoperative or postoperative Hgb level was less than 6 g/dL.[17] In addition, individuals with underlying cardiovascular disease and a Hgb level of less than 10 g/dL had a higher mortality than patients without cardiovascular disease. These results suggested that patients with underlying cardiovascular disease were less tolerant of anemia.

Several large retrospective analyses also examined the association between anemia and perioperative morbidity and mortality. One study of more than 310,000 hospitalized patients 65 years of age or older undergoing major noncardiac surgery found mild preoperative anemia to be associated with increased 30-day mortality and cardiovascular morbidity.[18] Similar findings were identified in 227,000 patients who underwent major noncardiac surgery as part of the American College of Surgeons' National Surgical Quality Improvement Program database.[19]

In the outpatient setting, anemia has also been associated with lower quality of life in patients with malignancy. Although fatigue is often multifactorial in cancer patients, it is extremely common in individuals with chemotherapy-induced anemia, occurring in more than 75% of patients in one study.[20] Decreased Hgb levels were correlated with increased fatigue and reduced measures of quality of life. Other studies suggested improvements in Hgb levels were associated with decreased fatigue score in patients with malignancy.[8]

CLINICAL TRIALS

There have been more than 25 clinical trials performed in adults and pediatric patients comparing liberal and restrictive RBC transfusion in greater than 12,000 patients.[21,22] These trials have been performed in many different clinical settings, including intensive care unit (ICU) patients; those undergoing cardiac, orthopedic, and other surgery; patients suffering from gastrointestinal bleeding or sepsis; and other settings. Liberal transfusion refers to RBC transfusion at higher Hgb triggers such as 9 or 10 g/dL. Restrictive transfusion refers to the use of lower Hgb transfusion triggers such as 7 or 8 g/dL. Although only 1 small trial has focused on surgical patients with malignancy, many studies have included cancer patients and these findings are relevant to their care. Relevant clinical trials have been performed in ICU patients including those with sepsis and abdominal malignancy, postoperative patients with cardiovascular risk factors, and patients with upper gastrointestinal bleeding. These trials are relevant in that they deal with common scenarios and complications in the treatment of malignancy. They are also important in that they were large, rigorously performed, and broke new ground that has resulted in a change in transfusion practice.

Intensive Care Unit and Sepsis

The Transfusion Requirement in Critical Care trial (TRICC) was the first to challenge the widely held view that a threshold of 10 g/dL was required to recover from acute life-threatening illness.[23] A total of 838 euvolemic intensive unit patients with a Hgb of less than 9 g/dL were randomly allocated to a 10 g/dL RBC transfusion threshold (liberal) group or a 7 g/dL RBC transfusion threshold (restrictive) group. The 30-day mortality was lower in patients in restrictive group (18.7%) than the 10 g/dL group (23.3%; $P = .1$) as were cardiovascular and pulmonary complications. The TRICC trial was the first to suggest that a 7 g/dL threshold was as safe and perhaps safer than a 10 g/dL threshold.

More recently, the Transfusion Requirements in Septic Shock (TRISS) trial, a randomized control trial in 1005 patients with septic shock in the ICU, found no difference in mortality or morbidity in individuals allocated to liberal (<9 g/dL) versus restrictive (<7 g/dL) transfusion strategies.[24] Consensus criteria for sepsis were used and RBC transfusions were given as single units of leukoreduced RBCs. Other outcomes, including the need for mechanical ventilation, vasopressors, renal replacement therapy, or other ischemic events, were also similar between the 2 groups. Among the enrolled patients, 7.5% had a history of hematologic malignancies and there were no differences between findings in this subgroup and the remainder of the cohort.

There are 3 trials evaluating RBC transfusion thresholds in pediatric populations. The largest trial was performed in 637 critically ill children cared for in pediatric ICUs at 19 centers.[25] Patients were enrolled with a Hgb level of less than 9.5 g/dL and randomly allocated to transfusion at 7 g/dL or 9.5 g/dL thresholds. The primary outcome of new or progressive multiple-organ dysfunction syndrome was similar between the 2 groups. Secondary outcomes, including transfusion reactions, respiratory and catheter-related infections, duration of stay, and mortality, were also not different between groups. Two smaller trials in premature infants that included neurocognitive outcomes have been published and a definitive trial (Transfusion of Prematures) is underway in this group of patients.[26]

In total, the findings of these trials in adult and pediatric ICUs have helped established practice recommendations for using a restrictive strategy (<7 g/dL) for RBC transfusion in critically ill patients without ischemic or congenital heart disease.

Bleeding

Patients with malignancy may have a more profound blood loss anemia related to a number of cancer-specific causes. Management of bleeding from a tumor can be complex and may be exacerbated by concomitant coagulopathy and/or thrombocy-topenia.[27] Coagulopathy occurs with increased frequency in patients with malignancy and can be owing to acquired inhibitors of coagulation, disseminated intravascular coagulation, or therapeutic anticoagulation to treat thromboembolism. Thrombocyto-penia is common in hematologic malignancies and may occur as a direct effect of bone marrow infiltration or a byproduct of chemotherapy.

Data on the management of transfusion in bleeding patients are from 2 clinical trials of upper gastrointestinal bleeding. The first study enrolled 921 patients in a trial comparing a 7 g/dL threshold (restrictive) with a 9 g/dL threshold (liberal).[28] At 6 weeks, 5% of the patients in the restrictive group died compared with 9% of the patients in the liberal group (hazard ratio, 0.55; 95% CI, 0.33–0.92; P = .02). The restrictive strategy was also associated with less rebleeding and congestive heart failure. An increased portal pressure gradient in the liberal group (P = .03) was hypothesized to explain the increased rate of rebleeding in the liberal transfusion group that included a signif-icant number of patients with cirrhosis. This trial was the first to report a statistically lesser mortality rate in patients in a restrictive RBC transfusion group.

Another recently published clinical trial assessed the effectiveness of transfusion strategies for acute upper gastrointestinal bleeding. The Transfusion in Gastrointes-tinal Bleeding (TRIGGER) trial, a pragmatic, cluster randomized feasibility trial random-ized patients to a 8 g/dL (restrictive) or 10 g/dL (liberal) transfusion threshold.[29] In a 6-month period, 936 patients were enrolled across 6 university hospitals in the United Kingdom. The cluster design led to rapid recruitment and high protocol adherence but a nonsignificant reduction in RBC transfusion in the restrictive arm. No differences in clinical outcomes were noted in this pilot trial in which 10% of enrolled subjects had a history of malignancy.

The findings of these trials in patients with upper gastrointestinal bleeding raises the possibility that hemodynamically stable patients with other sites of bleeding and who are without cardiovascular comorbidities or thrombocytopenia could be managed with a restrictive transfusion strategy safely.

Bleeding risk in relation to platelet transfusion thresholds has been well-studied in patients with malignancy; however, the optimal Hgb thresholds in thrombocytopenic patients are not known. Neither of these 2 clinical trials enrolled a significant number of patients who required platelet transfusions. Preclinical studies suggest that concom-itant anemia and thrombocytopenia may compound bleeding risk, and that hemostasis can be optimized in thrombocytopenic patients by maintaining a higher hematocrit.[30]

Two clinical trials examine RBC transfusion thresholds in patients with hematologic malignancies where thrombocytopenia is common. A pilot trial was performed in 60 pa-tients undergoing induction chemotherapy or stem cell transplantation.[31] Patients were randomly allocated to receive 2 units of RBCs when the Hgb concentration was less than 8 g/dL or 2 units of RBCs when the Hgb concentration was less than 12 g/dL. The main hypothesis was that there would be less bleeding and less need for platelet transfusions in the group with the higher transfusion threshold. The pilot demonstrated that such a trial was feasible but was not powered to detect clinical differences in the groups. The second trial, Transfusion of Red Cells in Hematopoietic Stem Cell Transplantation (TRIST), is enrolling patients undergoing hematopoietic stem cell transplantation, and compares transfusion thresholds of at 7 and 9 g/dL.[32] The results of this trial, which is in progress, will include quality of life in addition to clinical outcomes.

Postoperative Patients

In parallel with clinical trial data of bleeding patients, our understanding of best prac-tice in postoperative management of anemia comes from several studies of elderly patients with cardiovascular risk factors undergoing orthopedic surgery. Cancer patients who are candidates for surgical resection often undergo potentially life-saving procedures with the understanding that advanced age and cardiovascular comorbidities put them at increased risk of adverse outcomes as a result of significant blood loss.

The Functional Outcomes in Cardiovascular Patients Undergoing Surgical Hip Fracture Repair (FOCUS) trial enrolled elderly patients with underlying cardiovascular disease or risk factors who underwent surgical repair of hip fracture.[33] FOCUS compared a 10 g/dL transfusion threshold with an 8 g/dL or symptoms threshold. No difference was found in the primary outcome of death or inability to walk across a room unassisted; 35.2% in the liberal group and 34.7% in the restrictive group. There were also no differences in secondary outcomes including mortality at 60 days (liberal, 7.6% vs restrictive, 6.6%), infection, function, or duration of hospital stay. Furthermore, the composite outcome of acute myocardial infarction, unstable angina, or in-hospital mortality was not different in the liberal group (4.3%) and the restrictive group (5.2%). FOCUS was the first trial to provide evidence that patients with preexisting cardiovascular disease or risk factors could be safely managed postoperatively using a restrictive transfusion strategy.

The FOCUS trial was also significant in that it included functional status in postoperative patients as an outcome of different transfusion strategies. There was no difference in the ability to walk 10 feet or across a room without assistance at the 60-day evaluation. A systematic review of this trial and 5 others in patients with orthopedic fracture came to similar conclusions regarding the safety of restrictive transfusion practice.[34]

More recently, a small clinical trial of RBC transfusion practice enrolled 198 adult patients who underwent surgery for abdominal cancer (mostly gastrointestinal, pancreatic, or urogenital) and required postoperative intensive care.[35] Patients were randomized to a transfusion threshold of 7 g/dL (restrictive) or 9 g/dL (liberal) during their ICU stay; 21% and 42% of patients, respectively, were transfused in the 2 groups. The primary endpoint (death or severe complication at 30 days) occurred significantly more often in the restrictive group than in the liberal group (36% vs 20%). Several individual adverse outcomes also occurred more frequently with the restrictive strategy: 30-day mortality (23% vs 8%), 60-day mortality (24% vs 11%), cardiovascular complications (14% vs 5%), and abdominal infection (15% vs 5%).

The authors of this clinical trial suggested that maintaining a Hgb concentration of greater than 9 g/dL in postoperative cancer surgery patients is beneficial, although the study was limited by sample size and power. Their findings are contrary to the larger TRICC and TRISS trials in patients in the ICU, and the FOCUS trial in postoperative patients, which favored restrictive transfusion. In addition, a systematic review of clinical trials reporting data on in-hospital infections found a reduced risk among patients transfused with restrictive versus liberal transfusion strategies (risk ratio, 0.88; 95% CI, 0.78–0.99), and this finding was most striking in postoperative patients.[36] Although this apparent lower risk of infection may be reversed with publication of a clinical trial in cardiac surgery, it has nonetheless increased focus on postoperative complications of surgery as they relate to transfusion practice.[37] Additional studies are required to clarify differences in outcomes that may occur in surgical oncology patients.

Cardiovascular Events

Cardiovascular events occur with increased frequency in cancer patients than the general population as a result of the toxicity associated with therapies and the prevalence of cardiovascular risk factors in older individuals.[38] Patients with malignancy and coexistent coronary artery disease may be particularly prone to adverse outcomes–related cardiac ischemia, and whether they may benefit from a higher Hgb level remains debatable. In addition, patients with malignancy or those receiving chemotherapy are at greater risk of bleeding and may not be appropriate candidates for anticoagulation or antiplatelet agents in the setting of bleeding, thrombocytopenia, and/or coagulopathy.

In the absence of established treatments for myocardial ischemia, RBC transfusion may be beneficial by sustaining oxygen delivery to myocardial cells and decreasing myocardial oxygen demand. However, RBC transfusion could also worsen outcomes as a result of increased risk of circulatory overload or thrombogenicity with higher Hgb levels. Few clinical trials have focused on patients with malignancy, and transfusion strategies for the management of cardiovascular events in cancer patients can be extrapolated from the limited available data. Prior studies of cardiac surgery supported the safety of restrictive transfusion practice.[39,40] However, a more recent clinical trial of cardiac surgery patients found greater long-term mortality in the restrictive threshold group than in the liberal group (4.2% vs 2.6%; hazard ratio, 1.64; 95% CI, 1.00–2.67; $P = .045$).[37]

There have been 2 small clinical trials published that enrolled patients with acute coronary syndrome. Both trials compared transfusion triggers of 8 g/dL and 10 g/dL. In the Conservative Versus Liberal Red Cell Transfusion in Myocardial Infarction Trial (CRIT) trial, which included 45 patients, there was a higher incidence of congestive heart failure in the liberal group.[41] In the Myocardial Ischemia and Transfusion (MINT) trial in 110 patients, there was a trend toward fewer major cardiac events and deaths in the liberal group (7 deaths in restrictive strategy and 1 death in liberal strategy; $P = .03$).[42] Combining the 2 trials in acute coronary syndrome, there were 9 deaths in the restrictive group and 2 deaths in the liberal group. These trials are the first to signal that liberal transfusion might be superior to restrictive transfusion in the setting of acute coronary syndrome. However, these preliminary findings await a definitive answer in a large clinical trial.

TRANSFUSION ALTERNATIVES: ERYTHROPOIESIS-STIMULATING AGENTS

Recombinant human erythropoietin and other erythropoiesis-stimulating agents (ESAs) have been found to decrease the number of red blood transfusions in a variety of settings. In the US the Food and Drug Administration has approved erythropoietin for the treatment of:

i. Anemia in patients with chronic renal failure;
ii. Anemia in patients with human immunodeficiency virus infection receiving zidovudine;
iii. Highly selected cancer patients with anemia owing to myelosuppressive chemotherapy; and
iv. Patients with anemia who are at high risk for perioperative blood loss.

Metaanalyses of clinical trials of erythropoietin found significant decreases in the number of cancer patients receiving an RBC transfusion.[43,44] In patients with malignancy, ESAs were also considered a safe therapeutic option to improve functional status; however, early studies targeting a normal or high-normal Hgb levels had increased rates of thromboembolism and tumor progression.[45–49] Therefore, current guidelines for ESAs in cancer patients suggest they be used only in patients receiving chemotherapy and in those receiving palliative rather than curative treatment.[4] ESAs are not recommended currently for anemic cancer patients who are not receiving myelosuppressive chemotherapy or who have curable disease. In addition, guidelines recommend using ESA therapy only for patients with Hgb levels of less than 10 g/dL and optimizing iron status before ESA treatment.[7] However, a significant proportion of patients with malignancy do not achieve a hematologic response to ESA and functional iron deficiency is an important cause of ESA unresponsiveness.[50] There are few randomized studies on the use of ESAs to prevent or treat cancer associated anemia in children, and available data are limited by small sample size, study design, and heterogeneity in patient populations. Additional studies testing alternate dosing regimens may provide further data and clarify the potential benefits and toxicities associated with ESAs in adult and pediatric populations.

CLINICAL GUIDELINES

For many decades, the decision to transfuse RBCs was based on the "10/30 rule": transfusion was used to maintain a blood Hgb level of greater than 10 g/dL and a hematocrit of greater than 30%. Since that time, a large body of clinical trial evidence has been generated, resulting in the publication of multiple society guidelines for RBC transfusion in different settings.[9] Although clinical trial data focusing on patients with malignancy remains forthcoming, we emphasize available clinical trial data, because these provide the best evidence to guide transfusion decision making.

Published RBC transfusion guidelines addressed 4 questions that include the scope of both pediatric and adult patients with malignancy[9]:

1. In hospitalized, hemodynamically stable patients, at which Hgb concentration should a decision to transfuse RBCs be considered?
2. In hospitalized, hemodynamically stable patients with preexisting cardiovascular disease, at what Hgb concentration should a decision to transfuse RBCs be considered?
3. In hospitalized, hemodynamically stable patients with the acute coronary syndrome, at what Hgb concentration should an RBC transfusion be considered?
4. In hospitalized, hemodynamically stable patients, should transfusion be guided by symptoms rather than Hgb concentration?

Recommendations were based on a systematic review of the literature of clinical trials, and grading of the evidence.

In general, society guidelines recommended restrictive transfusion defined as 7 to 8 g/dL thresholds. The strongest recommendations are in the settings where there is direct clinical trial evidence including adult and pediatric ICU patients and orthopedic surgery patients undergoing hip fracture repair. The guidelines recommend 7 g/dL in ICU patients because that threshold was used in these trials, whereas 8 g/dL was used in surgery trials. The guidelines also recommend 8 g/dL threshold in patients with underlying cardiovascular disease, but acknowledge that only 1 trial has addressed this patient group. The guidelines make no specific recommendation in patients with acute coronary syndromes because there is no high-quality evidence in this patient population. Finally, the committee also advised using clinical symptoms to guide transfusion decisions, but these recommendations were judged to be based on low quality evidence and only received a weak recommendation because only 1 trial incorporated symptoms in the RBC transfusion decision-making process.

FUTURE STUDIES

Randomized, controlled clinical trials and other studies investigating optimal RBC transfusion thresholds are required to provide clinicians with evidence to guide its use in the setting of malignancy. Future studies should measure the impact of transfusion practice on several endpoints, including:

1. Quality of life and functional status of both inpatients and outpatients;
2. Impact on immunity and infection;
3. Bleeding events, especially in thrombocytopenic patients;
4. Neurocognitive development in pediatric populations; and
5. Survival and/or recurrence of disease.[51]

For cancer patients, the transfusion threshold and target Hgb that translate into optimal balance of risk and benefit in relation to quality of life and clinical outcomes remain unknown. It is possible that a higher Hgb target might lead to an improvement in quality of life in cancer patients, despite the negative impact that greater transfusion may have in regard to time commitment, potential for immunosuppression and infection, or possible transfusion reaction.

SUMMARY

The preponderance of clinical trial evidence supports using a restrictive transfusion strategy (7–8 g/dL) in most medical and surgical patients. However, additional studies are needed to understand best practice in the management of acute and chronic anemia in cancer patients with a focus on quality of life in addition to clinical outcomes.

REFERENCES

1. Ludwig H, van Belle S, Barrett-Lee P, et al. The European cancer anaemia survey (ECAS): a large, multinational, prospective survey defining the prevalence, incidence, and treatment of anaemia in cancer patients. Eur J Cancer 2004; 40(15):2293–306.
2. Maccio A, Madeddu C, Gramignano G, et al. The role of inflammation, iron, and nutritional status in cancer-related anemia: results of a large, prospective, observational study. Haematologica 2015;100(1):124–32.
3. Roy CN, Andrews NC. Anemia of inflammation: the hepcidin link. Curr Opin Hematol 2005;12(2):107–11.
4. Rodgers GM 3rd, Becker PS, Blinder M, et al. Cancer- and chemotherapy-induced anemia. J Natl Compr Canc Netw 2012;10(5):628–53.
5. Groopman JE, Itri LM. Chemotherapy-induced anemia in adults: incidence and treatment. J Natl Cancer Inst 1999;91(19):1616–34.
6. Michon J. Incidence of anemia in pediatric cancer patients in Europe: results of a large, international survey. Med Pediatr Oncol 2002;39(4):448–50.
7. Gilreath JA, Stenehjem DD, Rodgers GM. Diagnosis and treatment of cancer-related anemia. Am J Hematol 2014;89(2):203–12.
8. Birgegard G. Managing anemia in lymphoma and multiple myeloma. Ther Clin Risk Manag 2008;4(2):527–39.
9. Carson JL, Grossman BJ, Kleinman S, et al. Red blood cell transfusion: a clinical practice guideline from the AABB*. Ann Intern Med 2012;157(1):49–58.
10. Killick SB, Carter C, Culligan D, et al. Guidelines for the diagnosis and management of adult myelodysplastic syndromes. Br J Haematol 2014;164(4):503–25.

11. Vallet B, Adamczyk S, Barreau O, et al. Physiologic transfusion triggers. Best Pract Res Clin Anaesthesiol 2007;21(2):173–81.
12. Pinchon DJ, Stanworth SJ, Doree C, et al. Quality of life and use of red cell transfusion in patients with myelodysplastic syndromes. A systematic review. Am J Hematol 2009;84(10):671–7.
13. Goodnough LT, Levy JH, Murphy MF. Concepts of blood transfusion in adults. Lancet 2013;381(9880):1845–54.
14. Vamvakas EC. Transfusion-associated cancer recurrence and postoperative infection: meta-analysis of randomized, controlled clinical trials. Transfusion 1996;36(2):175–86.
15. Vamvakas EC, Blajchman MA. Transfusion-related immunomodulation (TRIM): an update. Blood Rev 2007;21(6):327–48.
16. Carson JL, Duff A, Poses RM, et al. Effect of anaemia and cardiovascular disease on surgical mortality and morbidity. Lancet 1996;348(9034):1055–60.
17. Carson JL, Noveck H, Berlin JA, et al. Mortality and morbidity in patients with very low postoperative Hb levels who decline blood transfusion. Transfusion 2002; 42(7):812–8.
18. Wu WC, Schifftner TL, Henderson WG, et al. Preoperative hematocrit levels and postoperative outcomes in older patients undergoing noncardiac surgery. JAMA 2007;297(22):2481–8.
19. Musallam KM, Tamim HM, Richards T, et al. Preoperative anaemia and postoperative outcomes in non-cardiac surgery: a retrospective cohort study. Lancet 2011;378(9800):1396–407.
20. Vogelzang NJ, Breitbart W, Cella D, et al. Patient, caregiver, and oncologist perceptions of cancer-related fatigue: results of a tripart assessment survey. The Fatigue Coalition. Semin Hematol 1997;34(3 Suppl 2):4–12.
21. Carson JL, Carless PA, Hebert PC. Transfusion thresholds and other strategies for guiding allogeneic red blood cell transfusion. Cochrane Database Syst Rev 2012;(4):CD002042.
22. Holst LB, Petersen MW, Haase N, et al. Restrictive versus liberal transfusion strategy for red blood cell transfusion: systematic review of randomised trials with meta-analysis and trial sequential analysis. BMJ 2015;350:h1354.
23. Hebert PC, Wells G, Blajchman MA, et al. A multicenter, randomized, controlled clinical trial of transfusion requirements in critical care. Transfusion Requirements in Critical Care Investigators, Canadian Critical Care Trials Group [see comments]. N Engl J Med 1999;340(6):409–17.
24. Holst LB, Haase N, Wetterslev J, et al. Lower versus higher hemoglobin threshold for transfusion in septic shock. N Engl J Med 2014;371(15):1381–91.
25. Lacroix J, Hebert PC, Hutchison JS, et al. Transfusion strategies for patients in pediatric intensive care units. N Engl J Med 2007;356(16):1609–19.
26. Kirpalani H, Whyte RK, Andersen C, et al. The premature infants in need of transfusion (PINT) study: a randomized, controlled trial of a restrictive (low) versus liberal (high) transfusion threshold for extremely low birth weight infants. J Pediatr 2006;149(3):301–7.
27. Mannucci PM. Overview of bleeding in cancer patients. Pathophysiol Haemost Thromb 2003;33(Suppl 1):44–5.
28. Villanueva C, Colomo A, Bosch A, et al. Transfusion strategies for acute upper gastrointestinal bleeding. N Engl J Med 2013;368(1):11–21.
29. Jairath V, Kahan BC, Gray A, et al. Restrictive versus liberal blood transfusion for acute upper gastrointestinal bleeding (TRIGGER): a pragmatic, open-label, cluster randomised feasibility trial. Lancet 2015;386(9989):137–44.

30. Valeri CR, Cassidy G, Pivacek LE, et al. Anemia-induced increase in the bleeding time: implications for treatment of nonsurgical blood loss. Transfusion 2001;41(8): 977–83.
31. Webert KE, Cook RJ, Couban S, et al. A multicenter pilot-randomized controlled trial of the feasibility of an augmented red blood cell transfusion strategy for patients treated with induction chemotherapy for acute leukemia or stem cell transplantation. Transfusion 2008;48(1):81–91.
32. Tay J, Tinmouth A, Fergusson D, et al. Transfusion of red cells in hematopoietic stem cell transplantation (TRIST): study protocol for a randomized controlled trial. Trials 2011;12:207.
33. Carson JL, Terrin ML, Noveck H, et al. Liberal or restrictive transfusion in high-risk patients after hip surgery. N Engl J Med 2011;365(26):2453–62.
34. Brunskill SJ, Millette SL, Shokoohi A, et al. Red blood cell transfusion for people undergoing hip fracture surgery. Cochrane Database Syst Rev 2015;(4):CD009699.
35. de Almeida JP, Vincent JL, Galas FR, et al. Transfusion requirements in surgical oncology patients: a prospective, randomized controlled trial. Anesthesiology 2015;122(1):29–38.
36. Rohde JM, Dimcheff DE, Blumberg N, et al. Health care-associated infection after red blood cell transfusion: a systematic review and meta-analysis. JAMA 2014; 311(13):1317–26.
37. Murphy GJ, Pike K, Rogers CA, et al. Liberal or restrictive transfusion after cardiac surgery. N Engl J Med 2015;372(11):997–1008.
38. Yeh ET, Tong AT, Lenihan DJ, et al. Cardiovascular complications of cancer therapy: diagnosis, pathogenesis, and management. Circulation 2004;109(25): 3122–31.
39. Bracey AW, Radovancevic R, Riggs SA, et al. Lowering the hemoglobin threshold for transfusion in coronary artery bypass procedures: effect on patient outcome. Transfusion 1999;39(10):1070–7.
40. Hajjar LA, Vincent JL, Galas FR, et al. Transfusion requirements after cardiac surgery: the TRACS randomized controlled trial. JAMA 2010;304(14):1559–67.
41. Cooper HA, Rao SV, Greenberg MD, et al. Conservative versus liberal red cell transfusion in acute myocardial infarction (the CRIT randomized pilot study). Am J Cardiol 2011;108(8):1108–11.
42. Carson JL, Brooks MM, Abbott JD, et al. Liberal versus restrictive transfusion thresholds for patients with symptomatic coronary artery disease. Am Heart J 2013;165(6):964–71.
43. Rizzo JD, Brouwers M, Hurley P, et al. American Society of Clinical Oncology/American Society of Hematology clinical practice guideline update on the use of epoetin and darbepoetin in adult patients with cancer. J Clin Oncol 2010; 28(33):4996–5010.
44. Seidenfeld J, Piper M, Flamm C, et al. Epoetin treatment of anemia associated with cancer therapy: a systematic review and meta-analysis of controlled clinical trials. J Natl Cancer Inst 2001;93(16):1204–14.
45. Corwin HL, Gettinger A, Fabian TC, et al. Efficacy and safety of epoetin alfa in critically ill patients. N Engl J Med 2007;357(10):965–76.
46. Littlewood TJ, Bajetta E, Nortier JW, et al. Effects of epoetin alfa on hematologic parameters and quality of life in cancer patients receiving nonplatinum chemotherapy: results of a randomized, double-blind, placebo-controlled trial. J Clin Oncol 2001;19(11):2865–74.
47. Hedley BD, Allan AL, Xenocostas A. The role of erythropoietin and erythropoiesis-stimulating agents in tumor progression. Clin Cancer Res 2011;17(20):6373–80.

48. Bennett CL, Silver SM, Djulbegovic B, et al. Venous thromboembolism and mortality associated with recombinant erythropoietin and darbepoetin administration for the treatment of cancer-associated anemia. JAMA 2008;299(8):914–24.

49. Gabrilove JL, Cleeland CS, Livingston RB, et al. Clinical evaluation of once-weekly dosing of epoetin alfa in chemotherapy patients: improvements in hemoglobin and quality of life are similar to three-times-weekly dosing. J Clin Oncol 2001;19(11): 2875–82.

50. Bokemeyer C, Aapro MS, Courdi A, et al. EORTC guidelines for the use of erythropoietic proteins in anaemic patients with cancer: 2006 update. Eur J Cancer 2007;43(2):258–70.

51. Spitalnik SL, Triulzi D, Devine DV, et al. 2015 proceedings of the national heart, lung, and blood institute's state of the science in transfusion medicine symposium. Transfusion 2015;55(9):2282–90.

Platelet Transfusions in Patients with Hypoproliferative Thrombocytopenia

Conclusions from Clinical Trials and Current Controversies

Gemma L. Crighton, BHB, MBChB[a,b,c], Lise J. Estcourt, MB, BChir[d],
Erica M. Wood, MBBS[a,e], Simon J. Stanworth, MD, DPhil[d],*

KEYWORDS

- Platelet transfusion • Thrombocytopenia • Bleeding • Acute leukemia
- Hematopoietic stem cell transplantation • Chemotherapy

KEY POINTS

- A uniform prophylactic platelet transfusion strategy for all patients with thrombocytopenia is not appropriate.
- Patients may have significant bleeding at platelet counts of greater than 10×10^9/L and should be assessed and managed on clinical grounds, not platelet count alone.
- Platelet count is not the only factor that contributes to a patient's propensity to bleed.
- Patients with acute leukemia should receive prophylactic platelet transfusions when their platelet count is less than 10×10^9/L to prevent clinical bleeding.
- Greater consistency in the assessment and documentation of bleeding across transfusion trials is essential to support comparisons of outcomes between studies.

Disclosure Statement: None.
[a] Department of Epidemiology and Preventive Medicine, The Alfred Centre, Monash University, Level 6, 99 Commercial Road, Melbourne, Victoria, 3181, Australia; [b] Australian Red Cross Blood Service, 100-154 Batman Street, West Melbourne, Victoria, 3003, Australia; [c] Royal Children's Hospital, Department of Haematology, 50 Flemington Road, Parkville, Victoria, 3052, Australia; [d] Radcliffe Department of Medicine, National Health Service Blood and Transplant, Oxford University Hospitals NHS Trust, John Radcliffe Hospital, University of Oxford, Oxford OX3 9BQ, UK; [e] Monash Health, Department of Haematology, 246 Clayton Road, Clayton, Victoria, 3168, Australia
* Corresponding author.
E-mail address: simon.stanworth@nhsbt.nhs.uk

Hematol Oncol Clin N Am 30 (2016) 541–560
http://dx.doi.org/10.1016/j.hoc.2016.01.002
0889-8588/16/$ – see front matter

INTRODUCTION

Duke[1] reported the first description of bleeding in the setting of thrombocytopenia, which improved after blood transfusion and recurred when the platelet count decreased. Up to 70% of patients with hematologic malignancy will have clinically significant bleeding (World Health Organization [WHO] grade 2 or higher) and up to 10% will have severe or life-threatening bleeding.[2]

Patients have a tendency to develop bleeding symptoms as their platelet counts decrease, and major bleeding occurs more frequently at platelet counts of less than $10 \times 10^9/L$.[2,3] However, many patients with severe thrombocytopenia do not develop clinically significant bleeding.[4,5] Conversely, major and even fatal bleeding is well-recognized to occur at platelet counts of greater than $10 \times 10^9/L$.[2,4–7]

In early leukemia studies, bleeding as a result of thrombocytopenia was a major contributing factor to mortality rates.[8] Platelet transfusions helped to decrease the incidence of death attributable to bleeding[8,9] and today mortality as a result of thrombocytopenia-related bleeding is exceedingly rare[2] (**Table 1**). Platelet transfusions have become an important adjunctive therapy and led to improved patient survival. They have also supported delivery of more intensive chemotherapy regimens.[8–10]

Platelet concentrates are the second most commonly prescribed blood product after red blood cells (RBC)[11] and hematooncology patients are the largest users of platelet concentrates.[12–14] Platelet transfusion rates are increasing; in the United States, more than 2 million platelet units were transfused in 2011, a 7.3% increase compared with 2008.[14] Platelet transfusions may be given therapeutically, to treat bleeding when thrombocytopenia or abnormal platelet function are contributing factors, but are more frequently given prophylactically, in efforts to avert bleeding before a procedure or when the platelet count falls below a certain threshold.[12,15,16] Many patients with platelet counts of less than $10 \times 10^9/L$ will not have clinically significant bleeding, and therefore many platelet transfusions may be being given unnecessarily.

METHODS

This review provides an update of the literature and some of the challenges raised by a very recent update of a Cochrane systematic review.[17] The methodology of this update has been described elsewhere; in brief, searching for platelet transfusion trials multiple datasets was undertaken. Eligible trials were identified and data abstracted, alongside an assessment of risk of bias. The update of an earlier Cochrane review[18] aimed to determine whether therapeutic-only platelet transfusions were as effective and safe as prophylactic platelet transfusions in patients with hematologic disorders undergoing cytotoxic chemotherapy or hematopoietic stem cell transplantation (HSCT).[17] Seven randomized controlled trials (RCTs) met the predefined selection criteria (one is still ongoing), leaving a total of 6 eligible trials and a total of 1195 participants. These trials were conducted over a 35-year time period. Five studies contained separate data for each arm and were able to be critically appraised. Only 1 study was deemed to be at low risk of bias.[4]

MAIN FINDINGS FOR REVIEW

For the systematic review's primary outcome (number of patients with ≥ 1 bleeding episode within 30 days) significant heterogeneity was noted ($I^2 = 88\%$).[17] This heterogeneity may reflect in part the different methodology and grading systems used to analyze and categorize bleeding in the individual studies. Four studies in the review[4,5,19,20] reported clinically significant bleeding events and all showed a similar effect: higher rates of bleeding in participants receiving therapeutic-only platelet transfusions. Major differences were noted between studies, including platelet transfusion indications, RBC transfusion policy, and study endpoints, as well as classification of bleeding events. Individual studies also reported bleeding outcomes over different time periods and used different units of analysis. For these reasons a metaanalysis was unable to be performed.[17]

Time to first bleeding episode was reported by 2 studies[4,5] and again metaanalysis was unable to be performed because of heterogeneity ($I^2 = 90\%$).[17] Individually, both studies showed that time to first bleeding episode was shorter in patients receiving therapeutic-only platelet transfusions.[17] One study reported the number of days with clinically significant bleeding events per patient and this was statistically higher in the therapeutic-only transfusion group.[4]

Owing to low mortality rates and rates of WHO grade 3 and 4 bleeding, there was insufficient evidence to determine whether there was any difference between platelet transfusion strategies for these outcomes.[17] Three studies[4,5,20] reported higher numbers of patients with WHO grade 3 or 4 bleeding events in the therapeutic-only transfusion group; however, a significant difference was not demonstrated, reflecting the rarity of this outcome.[17]

RECENT TRIALS

The systematic review included the results of 2 recent, large, multicenter RCTs; the Trial of Prophylactic versus No-Prophylactic Platelet Transfusions (TOPPS) and the trial by Wandt and colleagues.[4,5] Bleeding events were graded and reported differently in the trials; each trial used their own modification of the WHO bleeding scale and the same bleeding event would have been classified differently between studies[4,5] (**Table 2**). TOPPS reported that WHO grade 2 to 4 bleeding events occurred in 50% of patients in the therapeutic-only platelet transfusion group compared with 43% in the prophylaxis group; $P = .06$ for noninferiority, indicating that a therapeutic-only strategy was noninferior to prophylactic platelet transfusions.[4] Analysis of TOPPS data by the systematic review found that although there seemed to be an increased risk of bleeding events with a therapeutic-only transfusion policy, the 95% CI crossed 1.0 (relative risk [RR], 1.17; 95% CI, 0.99–1.39).[17] In the study by Wandt and colleagues,[5] therapeutic-only transfusions were associated with an increased risk of WHO grade 2 to 4 bleeding events per treatment cycle ($P<.0001$).

DISEASE AND TREATMENT CATEGORY

Many factors can affect a patient's bleeding susceptibility, including disease and treatment category, genetic predisposition, and concurrent medications. Different platelet RCTs have used different disease and treatment cohorts: acute leukemia patients receiving induction or consolidation chemotherapy,[6,7,21–23] HSCT patients,[21,24] and both acute leukemia or HSCT patients[2,4,5,25,26] (**Table 3**).

RCTs and systematic reviews have indicated that bleeding rates differ between patient disease and treatment categories.[2,4,5,18,26] Lower bleeding rates are noted in patients during autologous HSCT than during chemotherapy or allogeneic HSCT.[2,18,24,26] Tinmouth and colleagues[26] reported minor bleeding in 56% of acute leukemia patients versus 18% for autologous HSCT patients, and major bleeding in 23.5% of leukemia patients compared with 2.6% in the autologous group. Slichter and colleagues[2] similarly reported lower rates of WHO grade 2 to 4 bleeding in patients receiving autologous/synergeic HSCT (57%) compared with those receiving

Table 1
Rates of clinically significant bleeding and death from bleeding in the platelet transfusion randomized, controlled trials

Trial	Total Patients (n)	Bleeding Scale	Bleeding Assessment and Rates of Bleeding	Deaths from Hemorrhage (n)
Therapeutic only vs prophylactic platelet transfusions				
Solomon et al,[62] 1978	31	Not defined	Not reported	0
Sintnicolaas et al,[63] 1982	12	Not defined	Not reported	0
Grossman et al,[20] 1980	100	Study specific Mild (not requiring active intervention) vs severe	*Mild* 86 (86%) · *Severe* 74 (74%)	14[e]
Murphy et al,[19] 1982	56	Study specific	*Clinically significant bleeding event* 21 bleeds from study enrollment until study closure (37.5%) 15 bleeds in the first 10 mo of the study (27%)	3
Wandt et al,[5] 2012	396	Modified WHO	WHO grade 2 Reported per treatment cycle · *Grade 3* 10 (2.5%) · *Grade 4* 18 (4.5%)	2
Stanworth et al,[4] 2013	600	Modified WHO	WHO grade 2 272 (45%) · *Grade 3* 5 (0.8%) · *Grade 4* 2 (0.3%)	0
Platelet dose				
Roy et al,[7] 1973	62	Study specific	*Minor*[a] 18 (29%) · *Major*[b] 7 (11%)	NR
Steffens et al,[64] 2002	54	Not reported	NR	NR
Sensébé et al,[33] 2005	101	WHO 1979[65]	*Hemorrhaging* 14 (14%) · *WHO grades 2–3* 5 (5%) · *Grade 4* NR	NR
Tinmouth et al,[26] 2004	111	Modified GIMEMA	*Minor* 33 (30%) · *Major* 10 (9%)	0

	N	Scale				
Heddle et al,[25] 2009	129	Modified WHO	WHO grade 2 56 (43%)	Grade 3 11 (8.5%)	Grade 4 3 (2.3%)	0
Slichter et al,[2] 2010	1351	Modified WHO	WHO grade 2 177 (13%)	Grade 3 24 (1.8%)	Grade 4 7 (0.5%)	1
Platelet trigger						
Heckman et al,[23] 1997	78	Ajani 1990[66]	Any bleeding event 72 (92%)	Significant bleeding event 24 (31%)		0
Rebulla et al,[6] 1997	255	Study specific GIMEMA scale	Major 53 (21%)			1
Zumberg et al,[24] 2002	159	Modified GIMEMA	Minor[c] 128 (8%)	Major[d] 25 (16%)		0
Diedrich et al,[21] 2005	166	WHO 1979[65]	WHO grade 2 19 (11%)	Grades 3–4 8 (4.8%)		1
Platelets vs other product						
Higby et al,[22] 1974	21	Study specific	Hemorrhage 13 (6%)	Serious bleeding 9 (4%)		0

Abbreviations: GIMEMA, Gruppo Italiano Malattie Ematologiche Dell'Adulto; NR, not reported; WHO, World Health Organization.
[a] Skin, mucous membranes of mouth, lips, gums, epistaxis.
[b] Genitourinary and Gastrointestinal tracts.
[c] Minor bleeding events (petechial, mucosal, and microscopic bleeding) as well as melena and hematemesis not requiring red blood cell (RBC) transfusion.
[d] Major bleeding events (gross hematuria, any bleed requiring RBC), retinal bleeding, or central nervous system bleeding.
[e] Bacterial and/or fungal sepsis were a contributing factor in 8 of these deaths.
Data from Refs.[2,4–7,19–26,33,62–66]

Table 2
Platelet transfusion randomized, controlled trials with study adaptations of the WHO bleeding scale

	WHO Grade 3	WHO Grade 4

Heddle et al,[25] 2009	Oral, nasal, skin, musculoskeletal, GI, GU, pulmonary, invasive sites, other
	Bleeding requiring RBC transfusion specifically for support of bleeding within 24 hours of onset.
	Retinal[b]
	  —
	CNS
	  —
		Any source
		Fatal bleeding
		Debilitating bleeding
		Retinal
		  Retinal bleeding with visual impairment
		CNS
		  Nonfatal CNS bleeding

Wandt et al,[5] 2012	Oral, nasal, skin, musculoskeletal, GI, GU, pulmonary, invasive sites, other
	Bleeding necessitating RBC transfusion over routine needs within 24 hours
	Retinal
	  Routine fundoscopy without visual impairment
	CNS
		Oral, nasal, skin, musculoskeletal, GI, GU, pulmonary, invasive sites, other
		Bleeding necessitating RBC transfusion and associated with severe hemodynamic instability necessitating ICU
		Retinal
		  Bleeding with visual impairment proven by fundoscopy
		CNS
		  Fatal or nonfatal CNS bleeding

Slichter et al,[2] 2010	Oral, nasal, skin, musculoskeletal, GI, GU, pulmonary
	Bleeding requiring RBC transfusion over routine transfusion needs[a]
	Body cavity
	  Grossly bloody body cavity fluids and organ dysfunction with symptoms, and/or need to intervene (eg, to aspirate).
	Retinal[b]
	  CNS
	  LP with visible blood in absence of symptoms, and nontraumatic tap
		Any site
		Fatal bleeding
		Bleeding associated with severe hemodynamic instability and requiring RBC transfusion over routine transfusion needs
		Retinal
		  Bleeding with visual impairment
		CNS
		  CNS symptoms with nontraumatic bloody LP
		  CNS bleeding on imaging with or without dysfunction

Stanworth et al,[4] 2013	Oral, nasal, skin, musculoskeletal, GI, GU, pulmonary, invasive sites	Any site
	Bleeding requiring RBC transfusion specifically for support of bleeding within 24 hours of onset and without hemodynamic instability	Fatal bleeding any source
		Debilitating bleeding
		Bleeding associated with hemodynamic instability
	Body cavity	
	Bleeding in body cavity fluids grossly visible	
	Retinal bleeding[b]	Retinal bleeding
	—	Retinal bleeding and visual impairment
	CNS	CNS
	Cerebral bleeding noted on CT without neurologic signs and symptoms	Nonfatal cerebral bleeding with neurologic signs and symptoms

Abbreviations: CNS, central nervous system; CT, computed tomography; GI, gastrointestinal; GU, genitourinary; ICU, intensive care unit; LP, lumbar puncture; RBC, red blood cell; WHO, World Health Organization.

[a] RBC transfusion must be specifically related to treatment of bleeding within 24 hours of onset of bleeding.

[b] Retinal bleeding without visual impairment classified as WHO grade 2.

Data from Refs.[2,4,5,25]

Table 3
Platelet transfusion randomized controlled trials: inclusion and exclusion criteria

Trials	Inclusion Criteria	Exclusion Criteria
Therapeutic-only versus prophylactic transfusion trials		
Solomon et al,[62] 1978	Adults with AML	APML
Grossman et al,[20] 1980	Patients with amegakaryocytic thrombocytopenia	Refractory to platelet transfusions No longer candidate for aggressive therapy TCP not expected to last for >7 d
Murphy et al,[19] 1982	Pediatric patients Untreated acute leukemia	Not reported
Sintnicolaas et al,[63] 1982	Patients with acute leukemia and severe TCP	Not reported
Wandt et al,[5] 2012	AML Age 16–80 y AML trial participants, APML in complete remission Auto HSCT Age 16–65 y AML/ALL in first or second remission, non-Hodgkin lymphoma, Hodgkin lymphoma or multiple myeloma	APML (initial diagnosis) Platelet refractoriness Major bleeding with TCP when the reason for bleeding is still ongoing Plasmatic coagulation disorder Unable to consent
Stanworth et al,[4] 2013	Age ≥16 Hematologic malignancy received or receiving chemotherapy and/or HSCT Platelet count expected to be <50 for ≥5 d. Able to comply with treatment	APML WHO 3 bleeding or higher during treatment to date WHO 2 bleeding during current admission Inherited hemostatic or thrombotic disorder Antiplatelet or anticoagulants HLA antibodies Pregnant Prior randomization in this trial

Platelet dose studies

Study	Inclusion criteria	Exclusion criteria
Roy et al,[7] 1973	Pediatric hospitalized patients Acute leukemia Platelet count ≤25 × 10^9/L No active bleeding in previous 5 d	Not reported
Steffens et al,[64] 2002	Patients >16 y AML or undergoing an allogeneic HSCT	HLA antibodies Cardiovascular disease unable to tolerate a volume load
Sensebé et al,[33] 2005	Patients with acute leukemia undergoing first line treatment or autologous HSCT without criteria impairing platelet efficiency	APML
Tinmouth et al,[26] 2004	Patients >16 y AML or ALL receiving induction chemotherapy or autologous HSCT	APML Active bleeding Abnormal coagulation tests (INR >1.5, APTT >5 s greater than normal, fibrinogen <1.0 mg/dL) History of bleeding diathesis History of ITP, platelet refractoriness, anticoagulants, antiplatelet agents, antifibrinolytics or desmopressin acetate.
Heddle et al,[25] 2009	Weight 40–100 kg Hypoproliferative TCP Platelet count expected to be <10 × 10^9/L for a minimum of 10 d Receiving treatment as an inpatient	APML History of ITP, TTP, HUS WHO grade 2 bleeding or higher at entry Requiring bedside leukoreduced platelets Pregnancy
Slichter et al,[2] 2010	Any age Weight 10–135 kg HSCT or chemotherapy for hematologic malignancy or solid tumors Expected to have platelet count ≤10 for 5 d PT or APTT ≤1.3 x normal Fibrinogen ≥100 mg/dL No previous platelet transfusions for TCP during the current hospital admission.	APML WHO grade 2 bleeding or higher Bedside platelet leukoreduction Platelet refractoriness within past 30 d Panel reactive HLA antibody level of ≥20% ITP or TTP/HUS Planned prophylactic platelet transfusion at >10 × 10^9/L Major surgery within 2 wk Antiplatelet medications Pregnancy Previous enrolment in PLADO trial

(continued on next page)

Table 3
(continued)

Trials	Inclusion Criteria	Exclusion Criteria
Platelet trigger studies		
Heckman et al,[23] 1997	Age ≥17y Acute leukemia (AML, ALL in relapse, acute undifferentiated leukemia or MDS transformed to AML) Induction chemotherapy or re-induction after relapse	APML Inherited clotting disorder or history of bleeding diathesis Uncontrolled infection or DIC at randomization Concomitant malignancy AIDS Platelet refractoriness
Rebulla et al,[6] 1997	Adolescents and adults (17–70 y) Newly diagnosed AML admitted to hospital during their first course of chemotherapy	APML or secondary AML Received a blood transfusion before diagnosis of AML
Zumberg et al,[24] 2002	Patients >2 y Allogeneic, MUD or autologous BMT	Bleeding disorder or coagulopathy Anticoagulation Acute hemorrhage within 1 wk of enrolment or within 1 wk of a fall in the platelet count to below 50×10^9/L Prior bladder irradiation Planned use of cyclophosphamide Platelet alloimmunization
Diedrich et al,[21] 2005	All ages Allogeneic HSCT	Bleeding disorder or coagulopathy
Platelets versus other product		
Higby et al,[22] 1974	Afebrile, thrombocytopenic, AML patients	Hematologic remission Bleeding or hemolysis

Abbreviations: AIDS, acquired immune deficiency syndrome; ALL, acute lymphocytic leukemia; AML, acute myeloid leukemia; APML, acute promyelocytic leukemia; APTT, activated partial thromboplastin time; BMT, bone marrow transplant; DIC, disseminated intravascular coagulation; HSCT, hematopoietic stem cell transplantation; HUS, hemolytic uremic syndrome; INR, International Normalized Ratio; ITP, immune thrombocytopenia; MDS, myelodysplastic syndrome; MUD, matched unrelated donor; PT, prothrombin time; TCP, thrombocytopenia; TTP, thrombotic thrombocytopenic purpura; WHO, World Health Organization.
Data from Refs.[2,4–7,19–26,33,62–64]

chemotherapy for hematologic malignancies (73%) or allogeneic HSCT (79%). A metaanalysis performed in the 2012 Cochrane review showed a significantly lower risk of bleeding for autologous HSCT patients compared with patients receiving chemotherapy or allogeneic HSCT (RR, 0.73; 95% CI, 0.65–0.82).[18] Lower rates of bleeding in the autologous HSCT group may relate to faster platelet count recovery after autologous HSCT than after induction chemotherapy or allogeneic HSCT.[27]

The Cochrane systematic review 2015[17] identified 2 studies[4,5] that compared therapeutic-only versus prophylactic platelet transfusions in patients receiving autologous HSCT. As before, metaanalysis was not performed because of considerable heterogeneity (I^2 = 90%)[17] (see **Table 2**). Results from TOPPS showed no evidence of difference in the number of clinically significant bleeding episodes between transfusion strategies (RR, 1.04; 95% CI, 0.85–1.28).[17,28] However, the results from Wandt and colleagues[5] indicated a significant difference between transfusion protocols (RR, 3.45; 95% CI, 1.66–7.17); study authors reported P = .0005.

The systematic review found no difference in the number of patients undergoing autologous HSCT who experienced severe or life-threatening bleeding; however, this was a rare event and the 95% CI of the metaanalysis was wide.[17] The review concluded there was inconclusive evidence in autologous HSCT patients as to whether a therapeutic-only transfusion policy was associated with increased rates of clinically significant bleeding. Variability was noted in baseline patient characteristics between studies with regard to underlying hematologic disease requiring HSCT.[17] In TOPPS, no patients received autologous HSCT for acute leukemia, whereas Wandt and colleagues[5] included 13 patients with acute leukemia. It is unknown whether the underlying disease necessitating transplantation has any impact on bleeding rates.

Ford and colleagues[29] review of 125 Jehovah's witnesses undergoing autologous HSCT without prophylactic platelet transfusions may provide additional insight into safety of therapeutic-only platelet transfusions, with the addition of specific patient blood management strategies. Patients received antifibrinolytics as an alternative to platelet transfusions when the platelet count was less than 30 × 10^9/L. The authors reported 2 WHO grade 2 bleeds, 1 grade 3 bleed, 1 grade 4 bleed, and no bleeding-associated mortalities.[29]

The 2015 Cochrane systematic review[17] identified 3 studies[4,5,19] that compared therapeutic-only versus prophylactic platelet transfusions in patients with acute leukemia and all reported increased bleeding rates in patients receiving therapeutic-only platelet transfusions.[17] Again, a metaanalysis for this outcome was unable to be performed because of the different study endpoints and units of analysis.[17] TOPPS and Wandt and colleagues[5] both reported statistically higher rates of WHO grade 2 to 4 bleeding in patients with acute leukemia using therapeutic-only platelet transfusions.[4] Murphy and colleagues[19] reported higher numbers of bleed per 100 patient-months in the therapeutic-only group, but did not provide comparative statistical analysis for this outcome. A post hoc analysis by Wandt and colleagues[30] demonstrated higher numbers of WHO grade 3 and 4 in patients receiving induction chemotherapy compared with consolidation chemotherapy. Stanworth and colleagues'[28] post hoc analysis of TOPPS reported 2 WHO grade 3 bleeds in patients receiving induction chemotherapy and no grade 3 or 4 bleeds in patients receiving consolidation chemotherapy. These studies suggest that patients receiving induction chemotherapy are at higher risk of bleeding with therapeutic-only platelet transfusions than those receiving consolidation chemotherapy. Neither study has reported rates of WHO grade 2 bleeding events between induction and consolidation chemotherapy groups. The available evidence supports the ongoing use of prophylactic platelet transfusions to patients with acute leukemia receiving chemotherapy.

The 2015 Cochrane systematic review[17] found 1 study[4] that compared therapeutic-only with prophylactic platelet transfusions in patients receiving allogeneic HSCT.[17] Although the number of patients with clinically significant bleeding was higher in the therapeutic-only group, this was not significant and higher patient numbers would be needed to confirm or refute this finding.[17] Post hoc statistical analysis from TOPPS found that chemotherapy/allogeneic HSCT patients in the therapeutic-only arm had the highest incidence of WHO grade 2 to 4 bleeding.[31] There is insufficient evidence to change current practice of prophylactically transfusing allogeneic HSCT patients.

The evidence indicates that the efficacy of prophylactic platelet transfusions differs between subgroups of patients with hematologic malignancies; there is little evidence that a prophylactic policy for platelet transfusion is a superior policy for patients receiving autologous HSCT. The findings also inform future research. Factors other than those addressed by administration of platelet transfusions are important in determining risk of bleeding. Because many patients continue to bleed despite prophylactic platelet transfusions, additional strategies are required to minimize bleeding in all patient groups. These issues are addressed elsewhere in this paper.

PLATELET DOSE

In the United States, Food and Drug Administration Standards state that more than 75% of platelet units must have a count of greater than 3.0×10^{11} equating to a dose of 0.04×10^{11} platelets per 75 kg adult.[32]

The 2012 Cochrane systematic review[18] identified 6 RCTs that compared different platelet doses for prophylactic transfusion. A lower platelet transfusion dose did not result in an increased risk of WHO grade 2 to 4 bleeding (RR, 1.02; 95% CI, 0.93–1.11).[18] This review included the Platelet Dose (PLADO) study, an RCT in which patients undergoing HSCT or chemotherapy for malignancy were randomized to low dose (1.1×10^{11} platelets per m^2 body surface area), medium dose (2.2×10^{11}), and high dose (4.4×10^{11}) platelet transfusion when their morning platelet count was 10×10^9/L or less. This study found that the prophylactic platelet transfusion dose had no effect on the incidence of bleeding. Lower doses decreased the number of platelet transfusions ($P<.001$) without comprising haemostasis.[2] However, post-transfusion platelet counts were higher in those receiving the higher platelet transfusion dose.[2] This finding has been confirmed in other trials and has been shown to translate to a longer interval between platelet transfusions.[10,33]

In the hospital in-patient setting, a low-dose platelet strategy is appropriate and effective at reducing clinically significant bleeding, but will result in more frequent platelet transfusions. A single adult platelet unit should be given and the patient's clinical condition and platelet count should be reassessed. In the outpatient setting it may be desirable to have a longer period between platelet transfusions to reduce the frequency of hospital visits for a patient and a higher platelet transfusion dose may allow reduced transfusion frequency.

PLATELET TRANSFUSION THRESHOLD

Gaydos and colleagues[3] first described the quantitative relationship between degree of thrombocytopenia and bleeding in leukemia patients receiving chemotherapy. At lower platelet counts the frequency, number of bleeding days and severity of bleeding events were increased. Grossly discernible hemorrhage rarely occurred at platelet counts of greater than 20×10^9/L, but rates increased when the count was 5 to 20×10^9/L and a steep increase occurred at platelet counts of less than 5×10^9/L. Although the authors concluded that a platelet threshold could not be determined, this study has frequently been cited as the origin of the platelet transfusion threshold of 20×10^9/L.[3]

The Platelet Transfusion Trigger Trial by Rebulla and colleagues[6] randomized adolescents and adults with a new diagnosis of acute myeloid leukemia (AML) receiving induction chemotherapy to a platelet transfusion threshold of less than 10×10^9/L compared with 20×10^9/L. No difference ($P = .41$) in bleeding endpoints was seen between patient groups and patients in the 10×10^9/L group received significantly fewer platelet transfusions.

The 2012 Cochrane systematic review[18] included 3 RCTs with different platelet count triggers and found no significant difference between platelet trigger and number of participants with clinically significant bleeding (RR, 1.35; 95% CI, 0.95–1.9).[18]

Currently, many hematology centers adopt the platelet transfusion trigger of 10×10^9/L. However, an even lower threshold of 5×10^9/L may be appropriate. Slichter and colleagues[2] demonstrated that bleeding occurred on 25% of study days when the platelet count was less than 5×10^9/L and 17% of the days when it was 6 to 80×10^9/L ($P<.001$). Observational studies have provided further evidence that patients may be safely managed by transfusing at a threshold of 5×10^9/L.[3,34–36] Ford and colleagues[29] reported their experience of performing autologous HSCT without platelet transfusions and reported no major bleeding events at platelet counts of less than 5×10^9/L.

Routine hematology analyzers are inaccurate at counting platelets in the setting of severe thrombocytopenia and frequently overestimate them.[37] Overestimation of the platelet count will potentially result in undertransfusion of platelets, particularly when the count is 5 to 10×10^9/L.[37] If patients are not bleeding, then a lower threshold may be appropriate. Higher thresholds of 20×10^9/L are frequently implemented by clinicians when a patient has concurrent headache, fever, infection, or coagulation disorders, or before invasive procedures.[38]

LIMITATIONS IN THE INTERPRETATION OF PLATELET TRANSFUSION TRIALS

Caution must be had in adopting a one size fits all approach because there may be important differences between patients enrolled in platelet RCTs and the patient seen in the clinic. Trials have specific inclusion and exclusion criteria, only including certain patient cohorts and treatment groups; therefore, results may not be generalizable to other patient groups. Patients enrolled in trials are likely to receive very attentive surveillance, with close monitoring of all bleeding events, new clinical symptoms and hematologic parameters (see **Tables 1** and **3**).

Platelet RCTs have been conducted in a variety of patient cohorts, namely, pediatric patients,[7,19] any age patient,[2,21] and only adolescents and adults.[4–6,21,23,25,26] (see **Table 3**). Roy and colleagues[7] found higher rates of bleeding in patients aged 0 to 4 years of age. Josephson's secondary analysis of the PLADO trial found children aged 0 to 5 years had a significantly higher risk of WHO grade 2 to 4 than those 19 years or older (86% vs 67%). Children from all age groups had more days of WHO grade 2 to 4 bleeding compared with adults.[39] Conclusions drawn from adult trials cannot be directly applied to pediatric patients.

Many trials exclude patients at highest risk of bleeding. Acute promyelocytic leukemia is associated with coagulopathy; hyperfibrinolysis and hemorrhagic complications are the most frequent cause of death in this group.[40] Many platelet RCTs exclude patients with acute promyelocytic leukemia[2,4,6,23,25,26,33]; only Wandt and colleagues[5] included acute promyelocytic leukemia patients once in complete remission. Patients with inherited hemostatic disorders and taking antiplatelet medications or anticoagulants are commonly excluded from trials.[2,5,21,23,24,26] Patients with platelet refractoriness are excluded in a number of trials.[2,5,23,24,26]

Careful attention must be taken when comparing bleeding events between studies. Bleeding assessment tools, the analysis and grading of bleeding events differ significantly between trials (see **Tables 1** and **2**). The WHO 1979 bleeding scale[41] provides a general classification system adopted for grading toxicities associated with cancer treatments: grade 0, no bleeding; grade 1, petechiae; grade 2, mild blood loss; grade 3, gross blood loss; and grade 4, debilitating blood loss.[41] These very nonspecific categories allow substantial interpretation by the clinician. Several trials have adapted the WHO bleeding scale with major differences between adaptations, particularly for grading of central nervous system and retinal bleeding events[2,4,5,25] (see **Table 2**). Grade 3 bleeding is frequently considered bleeding that necessitates RBC transfusion. However, RBC transfusion policies differ between studies; in TOPPS a hemoglobin of less than 90 g/L was used,[4] Wandt and colleagues transfused to maintain a hemoglobin of 80 g/L or greater, hemoglobin threshold was not reported by Heddle and colleagues,[25] and Slichter and colleagues[2] reported that RBC transfusion was indicated by local practice. Of platelet studies using the WHO scale or a modification; WHO grade 2 bleeding events were reported in 11% to 45% of patients,[2,4,21,25] WHO grade 3 events in 0.8% to 8.5%,[2,4,5,25] and WHO grade 4 bleeding events in 0.3% to 4.5%[2,4,5,25] (see **Table 1**).

Rebulla and colleagues[6] and the Gruppo Italiano Malattie Ematologiche Maligne dell'Adulto (GIMEMA) developed their own 8-point scale for bleeding assessment. RBCs were administered when the hemoglobin was less than 80 g/L.[6] In platelet transfusion RCTs using the GIMEMA scale or a modification thereof, minor bleeding rates were reported in 8% to 30%[24,26] and major bleeding rates in 9% to 21%.[6,24,26]

To analyze and compare bleeding events between studies a reliable and reproducible bleeding assessment tool is needed. The Bleeding Severity Measurement Scale will hopefully provide a valid and reliable measurement of bleeding.[42]

RISK FACTORS FOR BLEEDING ASIDE FROM PLATELET COUNT

Many patients have severe bleeding despite a platelet count of less than 10×10^9/L and sometimes at platelet counts of greater than 20×10^9/L.[4–6] Many studies have suggested that other factors contribute to a patient's tendency to bleed.[4–6]

The relationships between minor bleeding events, platelet counts, and more severe bleeding events have been reviewed by a number of trials. Although many trials do not specifically report WHO grade 1 bleeding as a study outcome,[2,4,5] this may be very important if it predicts more severe bleeding.[43] Webert and colleagues'[43] post hoc analysis of the Platelet Transfusion Trigger trial noted that the majority of severe bleeds were associated with bleeds of lesser severity in the preceding days. Patients with WHO grade 1 bleeding were 2.6 times more likely to experience WHO grades 2 to 4 bleeding on the next day. Friedmann and associates'[44] large retrospective review of thrombocytopenic patients, also reported a significant association between recent bleeding and the risk of severe hemorrhage. In contrast, post hoc statistical modeling from TOPPS found no evidence that minor bleeding predicted WHO grade 2 to 4 bleeding.[31] Stanworth and colleagues[31] did find that the number of days with a platelet count of less than 10×10^9/L was significantly associated with grade 2 to 4 bleeding and there was a significant association between platelet count on the previous day and hemorrhage. Similarly, Webert and colleagues[42] found that for every 1×10^9/L increase in platelet count there was a 4% decrease in the risk of grade 2 to 4 bleeding on the next day. In contrast, Friedmann's review found no relationship between first or lowest platelet count of the day and the risk of severe hemorrhage.[44] This may be owing to the retrospective nature of this study, that the analysis excluded WHO grade 2 bleeding events, and that the platelet count from the day before was the significant factor.

Fever has been identified by a number of studies as a potential risk factor for bleeding.[22,31,43] Early studies postulated that the association between bleeding and fever reflected the use of aspirin, which was historically given as an antipyretic.[44] Today aspirin and nonsteroidal antiinflammatory drugs are withheld, if possible, in hematooncology patients and patients taking these medications are excluded from clinical trials.[2,4,26] Webert and colleagues'[43] post hoc analysis found the risk of clinically significant bleeding was 3.35 times greater in the presence of clinical infection. In this study, platelet transfusions were given to patients in the 10×10^9/L trigger group when their platelet count was 10 to 20×10^9/L in the presence of fever.[6] Post hoc analysis of TOPPS found that patients with temperatures of 38°C or greater had the highest hazard of grade 2 to 4 bleeding.[31] In TOPPS, platelets were also given at physician's discretion; 18% of transfusions in the therapeutic-only group were for infection or when the patient was unwell compared with 11% in the prophylaxis group.[4] These results support a higher platelet threshold for patients who are febrile or have an infection. Older platelet transfusion guidelines support these findings and recommend a platelet transfusion trigger of 20×10^9/L in the presence of risk factors[45,46]; however, newer ones have not made recommendations supporting this practice.[47,48]

The TOPPS authors also found that female sex was significantly associated with WHO grade 2 to 4 bleeding.[31] Even when the authors removed menstrual bleeding data, female patients consistently had a higher risk of bleeding. The reason for this finding remains unclear.[31] Neither the reviews by Webert and colleagues[43] or Friedmann and colleagues[44] specifically analyzed sex as a risk factor for bleeding.

There may be a relationship between hemoglobin, RBC transfusion and risk of bleeding. In vitro studies by Escolar and colleagues[49] suggest that RBC are critical for maintenance of interactions between platelets and subendothelium. These interactions and bleeding times are improved consistently after RBC transfusion to patients with anemia and thrombocytopenia. Valeri and colleagues[50] reported that an acute decrease in hematocrit in normal individuals produced reversible platelet dysfunction and increased bleeding times, which normalized after RBC transfusion. In TOPPS, patients in the therapeutic-only transfusion group, who received RBC transfusion in the previous 3 days, were at increased risk of bleeding.[31] This increased risk of bleeding associated with recent RBC transfusion may reflect a recent history of significant anemia, necessitating the transfusion. Webert and colleagues[43] similarly reported that higher hemoglobin levels were associated with a delay in time to clinically significant bleeding. A 10 g/L increase in hemoglobin decreased the risk of clinically significant bleeding by 22% the next day.

Limitations in the post hoc and investigative analyses performed by Friedmann, Stanworth, and Webert include incomplete datasets, the retrospective nature of the studies, and time since the original study. However, they remain a valuable means to identify risk factors for bleeding and help stratify patients. Stable patients without risk factors may potentially be able to avoid prophylactic platelet transfusions.

HEMATOLOGIC DISEASE LINKED WITH BLEEDING

Hematologic diseases may be linked with bleeding dyscrasias. Abnormalities in platelet function may be associated with myelodysplastic syndrome and AML.[51] Severely thrombocytopenic patients with AML or myelodysplastic syndrome may have smaller platelets, lower immature platelet fractions, and substantially lower platelet surface expression of activated GPIIb/IIIa and GPIb than severely thrombocytopenic patients with immune thrombocytopenia.[52] Familial platelet disorders with predisposition to AML owing to RUNX1 mutations are associated with platelet dysfunction.[53]

Acquired von Willebrand disease is a rare bleeding disorder that is associated with lymphoproliferative disorders and myeloproliferative neoplasms.[54] It is characterized by structural and functional defects in von Willebrand factor.[54] Treatment involves controlling acute bleeding with von Willebrand factor–containing concentrates and attempting to obtain remission of the underlying disease by surgery, chemotherapy, radiotherapy, or immunosuppression.[54]

Patients with plasma cell dyscrasia such as multiple myeloma, Waldenstrom macroglobulinemia, monoclonal gammopathy of uncertain significance, and amyloidosis not infrequently develop bleeding symptoms such as purpura, epistaxis, or hematuria.[55] The implicated paraproteins interact with platelets and coagulation factors, causing multiple hemostatic abnormalities, including prolonged coagulation assays, factor deficiencies, and platelet dysfunction, resulting in bleeding.[55,56] Uremia and renal failure associated with advanced myeloma are additional risks for platelet dysfunction.

ANTIFIBRINOLYTICS

Tranexamic acid (TXA) is an antifibrinolytic that has been used to reduce the risk of death owing to hemorrhage in the trauma setting and reduce blood loss and the need for RBCs during surgery.[57,58] Shpilberg and colleagues'[59] small RCT of patients with AML receiving chemotherapy randomised participants to TXA or placebo and patients were only given platelets when bleeding occurred. Although the sample size was small, the authors found that, during consolidation chemotherapy, there was a significantly decreased bleeding tendency in the TXA group that resulted in lower platelet transfusion requirements. No difference in bleeding rates, severity, or platelet transfusion requirements were noted in the induction chemotherapy group.[59]

A 2013 Cochrane systematic review[60] evaluated the use of antifibrinolytics in patients with hematologic malignancies and found limited evidence for the use of antifibrinolytics in this cohort. Available data suggest that antifibrinolytics may reduce bleeding and therefore may be a useful adjunct to platelet transfusions.[60] The Trial to EvaluAte Tranexamic acid in Thrombocytopenia (TREATT) is an RCT currently recruiting patients that aims to examine whether giving TXA to patients receiving treatment for hematologic malignancies reduces the risk of bleeding or death and the need for platelet transfusions.[61]

SUMMARY

Platelet transfusions are an important adjunctive therapy in the management of hematology patients with hypoproliferative thrombocytopenia secondary to chemotherapy or HSCT. The systematic review concluded that overall prophylactic platelet transfusions seemed to reduce the number of bleeding events and days with clinically significant bleeding, therefore supporting the continued use of prophylactic platelet transfusions.[17] However, recent findings challenge the basis of a uniform policy of platelet transfusion prophylaxis for all patients. Individual patient, disease, and treatment characteristics increasingly need to be considered, and new guidelines need to reflect these implications. Studies report major bleeding occurs despite prophylactic platelet transfusions at platelet counts of greater than 10×10^9/L, indicating that patients should be managed clinically and not on the basis of platelet count alone.[4,5,20]

A better understanding of risk factors will identify patients at greater or lesser risk of bleeding, and hence more or less likely to experience benefit from platelet transfusions. Patients with acute leukemia receiving chemotherapy or undergoing allogeneic HSCT should continue to receive prophylactic platelet transfusions. There is no evidence that a prophylactic policy for platelet transfusion is superior for patients receiving autologous HSCT, and risk factors such as duration of severe thrombocytopenia and fever may be more relevant. Other research gaps include understanding donor factors and changes in platelet function, which are not captured by isolated measures of platelet count.

REFERENCES

1. Duke WW. The relation of blood platelets to hemorrhagic disease: description of a method for determining the bleeding time and coagulation time and report of three cases of hemorrhagic disease relieved by transfusion. JAMA 1910; 55(14):1185–92.
2. Slichter SJ, Kaufman RM, Assmann SF, et al. Dose of prophylactic platelet transfusions and prevention of hemorrhage. N Engl J Med 2010;362(7):600–13.
3. Gaydos LA, Freireich EJ, Mantel N. The quantitative relation between platelet count and hemorrhage in patients with acute leukemia. N Engl J Med 1962; 266:905–9.
4. Stanworth SJ, Estcourt LJ, Powter G, et al. A no-prophylaxis platelet-transfusion strategy for hematologic cancers. N Engl J Med 2013;368(19):1771–80.
5. Wandt H, Schaefer-Eckart K, Wendelin K, et al. Therapeutic platelet transfusion versus routine prophylactic transfusion in patients with haematological malignancies: an open-label, multicentre, randomised study. Lancet 2012;380(9850): 1309–16.
6. Rebulla P, Finazzi G, Marangoni F, et al. The threshold for prophylactic platelet transfusions in adults with acute myeloid leukemia. Gruppo Italiano Malattie Ematologiche Maligne dell'Adulto. N Engl J Med 1997;337(26):1870–5.
7. Roy AJ, Jaffe N, Djerassi I. Prophylactic platelet transfusions in children with acute leukemia: a dose response study. Transfusion 1973;13(5):283–90.
8. Hersh EM, Bodey GP, Nies BA, et al. Causes of death in acute leukemia: a ten-year study of 414 patients from 1954-1963. JAMA 1965;193:105–9.
9. Han T, Stutzman L, Cohen E, et al. Effect of platelet transfusion on hemorrhage in patients with acute leukemia. An autopsy study. Cancer 1966;19(12):1937–42.
10. Norol F, Bierling P, Roudot-Thoraval F, et al. Platelet transfusion: a dose-response study. Blood 1998;92(4):1448–53.
11. Poles D, et al. Bolton-Maggs PHB, editor. On behalf of the Serious Hazards of Transfusion (SHOT) Steering Group. The 2014 Annual SHOT Report. 2015.
12. Charlton A, Wallis J, Robertson J, et al. Where did platelets go in 2012? A survey of platelet transfusion practice in the North of England. Transfus Med 2014;24(4): 213–8.
13. Shehata N, Tinmouth A, Naglie G, et al. ABO-identical versus nonidentical platelet transfusion: a systematic review. Transfusion 2009;49(11):2442–53.
14. Whitaker BI. The 2011 National Blood Collection & Utilization Survey. 2011. Available at: http://www.hhs.gov/ash/bloodsafety/nbcus/2011-nbcus.pdf. Accessed August 28, 2015.
15. Bosch MA, Contreras E, Madoz P, et al. The epidemiology of blood component transfusion in Catalonia, Northeastern Spain. Transfusion 2011;51(1):105–16.

16. Freireich EJ, Kliman A, Gaydos LA, et al. Response to repeated platelet transfusion from the same donor. Ann Intern Med 1963;59:277–87.

17. Crighton GL, Estcourt LJ, Wood EM, et al. A therapeutic-only versus prophylactic platelet transfusion strategy for preventing bleeding in patients with haematological disorders after myelosuppressive chemotherapy or stem cell transplantation. Cochrane Database of Syst Rev 2015;(9):CD010981.

18. Estcourt L, Stanworth S, Doree C, et al. Prophylactic platelet transfusion for prevention of bleeding in patients with haematological disorders after chemotherapy and stem cell transplantation. Cochrane Database Syst Rev 2012;(5):CD004269.

19. Murphy S, Litwin S, Herring LM, et al. Indications for platelet transfusion in children with acute leukemia. Am J Hematol 1982;12(4):347–56.

20. Grossman L, Mangal A, Hislop TG, et al. Preliminary report on a randomized study of prophylactic vs. therapeutic platelet transfusions. International Society Blood Transfusion; 1980. p. 271. Abstract No. 1466. Warsaw.

21. Diedrich B, Remberger M, Shanwell A, et al. A prospective randomized trial of a prophylactic platelet transfusion trigger of 10 x 10(9) per L versus 30 x 10(9) per L in allogeneic hematopoietic progenitor cell transplant recipients. Transfusion 2005;45(7):1064–72.

22. Higby DJ, Cohen E, Holland JF, et al. The prophylactic treatment of thrombocytopenic leukemic patients with platelets: a double blind study. Transfusion 1974;14(5):440–6.

23. Heckman KD, Weiner GJ, Davis CS, et al. Randomized study of prophylactic platelet transfusion threshold during induction therapy for adult acute leukemia: 10,000/microL versus 20,000/microL. J Clin Oncol 1997;15(3):1143–9.

24. Zumberg MS, del Rosario ML, Nejame CF, et al. A prospective randomized trial of prophylactic platelet transfusion and bleeding incidence in hematopoietic stem cell transplant recipients: 10,000/L versus 20,000/microL trigger. Biol Blood Marrow Transplant 2002;8(10):569–76.

25. Heddle NM, Cook RJ, Tinmouth A, et al. A randomized controlled trial comparing standard- and low-dose strategies for transfusion of platelets (SToP) to patients with thrombocytopenia. Blood 2009;113(7):1564–73.

26. Tinmouth A, Tannock IF, Crump M, et al. Low-dose prophylactic platelet transfusions in recipients of an autologous peripheral blood progenitor cell transplant and patients with acute leukemia: a randomized controlled trial with a sequential Bayesian design. Transfusion 2004;44(12):1711–9.

27. Goncalves TL, Benvegnu DM, Bonfanti G. Specific factors influence the success of autologous and allogeneic hematopoietic stem cell transplantation. Oxid Med Cell Longev 2009;2(2):82–7.

28. Stanworth SJ, Estcourt LJ, Llewelyn CA, et al. Impact of prophylactic platelet transfusions on bleeding events in patients with hematologic malignancies: a subgroup analysis of a randomized trial. Transfusion 2014;54(10):2385–93.

29. Ford PA, Grant SJ, Mick R, et al. Autologous stem-cell transplantation without hematopoietic support for the treatment of hematologic malignancies in Jehovah's witnesses. J Clin Oncol 2015;33(15):1674–9.

30. Schaefer-Eckart K, Wendelin K, Pilz B, et al. Consolidation therapy is associated with significantly lower bleeding risk compared to induction therapy in patients with acute myeloid leukemia. Blood 2014;124(21):3686.

31. Stanworth SJ, Hudson CL, Estcourt LJ, et al. Risk of bleeding and use of platelet transfusions in patients with hematologic malignancies: recurrent event analysis. Haematologica 2015;100(6):740–7.

32. US Food and Drug Administration. Guidance for industry and FDA review staff: collection of platelets by automated methods. 2007. Available at: http://www.fda.gov/BiologicsBloodVaccines/GuidanceComplianceRegulatoryInformation/Guidances/Blood/ucm073382.htm. Accessed May 7, 2015.

33. Sensebé L, Giraudeau B, Bardiaux L, et al. The efficiency of transfusing high doses of platelets in hematologic patients with thrombocytopenia: results of a prospective, randomized, open, blinded end point (PROBE) study. Blood 2005; 105(2):862–4.

34. Gmur J, Burger J, Schanz U, et al. Safety of stringent prophylactic platelet transfusion policy for patients with acute leukaemia. Lancet 1991;338(8777):1223–6.

35. Slichter SJ, Harker LA. Thrombocytopenia: mechanisms and management of defects in platelet production. Clin Haematol 1978;7(3):523–39.

36. Sagmeister M, Oec L, Gmur J. A restrictive platelet transfusion policy allowing long-term support of outpatients with severe aplastic anemia. Blood 1999; 93(9):3124–6.

37. Segal HC, Briggs C, Kunka S, et al. Accuracy of platelet counting haematology analysers in severe thrombocytopenia and potential impact on platelet transfusion. Br J Haematol 2005;128(4):520–5.

38. Kretschmer V. Current trends in platelet transfusion – transfusion practices in Europe. Transfus Med Hemother 1996;23(Suppl 1):5–11.

39. Josephson CD, Granger S, Assmann SF, et al. Bleeding risks are higher in children versus adults given prophylactic platelet transfusions for treatment-induced hypoproliferative thrombocytopenia. Blood 2012;120(4):748–60.

40. Breen KA, Grimwade D, Hunt BJ. The pathogenesis and management of the coagulopathy of acute promyelocytic leukaemia. Br J Haematol 2012;156(1):24–36.

41. Miller AB, Hoogstraten B, Staquet M, et al. Reporting results of cancer treatment. Cancer 1981;47(1):207–14.

42. Webert KE, Arnold DM, Lui Y, et al. A new tool to assess bleeding severity in patients with chemotherapy-induced thrombocytopenia. Transfusion 2012; 52(11):2466–74 [quiz: 2465].

43. Webert K, Cook RJ, Sigouin CS, et al. The risk of bleeding in thrombocytopenic patients with acute myeloid leukemia. Haematologica 2006;91(11):1530–7.

44. Friedmann AM, Sengul H, Lehmann H, et al. Do basic laboratory tests or clinical observations predict bleeding in thrombocytopenic oncology patients? a reevaluation of prophylactic platelet transfusions. Transfus Med Rev 2002;16(1):34–45.

45. Schiffer CA, Anderson KC, Bennett CL, et al. Platelet transfusion for patients with cancer: clinical practice guidelines of the American Society of Clinical Oncology. J Clin Oncol 2001;19(5):1519–38.

46. British Committee for Standards in Haematology and Blood Transfusion Task Force. Guidelines for the use of platelet transfusions. Br J Haematol 2003; 122(1):10–23.

47. Kaufman RM, Djulbegovic B, Gernsheimer T, et al. Platelet transfusion: a clinical practice guideline from the AABB. Ann Intern Med 2015;162(3):205–13.

48. Nahirniak S, Slichter SJ, Tanael S, et al. Guidance on platelet transfusion for patients with hypoproliferative thrombocytopenia. Transfus Med Rev 2015; 29(1):3–13.

49. Escolar G, Garrido M, Mazzara R, et al. Experimental basis for the use of red cell transfusion in the management of anemic-thrombocytopenic patients. Transfusion 1988;28(5):406–11.

50. Valeri CR, Cassidy G, Pivacek LE, et al. Anemia-induced increase in the bleeding time: implications for treatment of nonsurgical blood loss. Transfusion 2001;41(8): 977–83.

51. Kantarjian H, Giles F, List A, et al. The incidence and impact of thrombocytopenia in myelodysplastic syndromes. Cancer 2007;109(9):1705–14.

52. Psaila B, Bussel JB, Frelinger AL, et al. Differences in platelet function in patients with acute myeloid leukemia and myelodysplasia compared to equally thrombocytopenic patients with immune thrombocytopenia. J Thromb Haemost 2011; 9(11):2302–10.

53. Jongmans MCJ, Kuiper RP, Carmichael CL, et al. Novel RUNX1 mutations in familial platelet disorder with enhanced risk for acute myeloid leukemia: clues for improved identification of the FPD/AML syndrome. Leukemia 2009;24(1):242–6.

54. Federici AB, Rand JH, Bucciarelli P, et al. Acquired von Willebrand syndrome: data from an international registry. Thromb Haemost 2000;84(2):345–9.

55. Zangari M, Elice F, Fink L, et al. Hemostatic dysfunction in paraproteinemias and amyloidosis. Semin Thromb Hemost 2007;33(4):339–49.

56. Perkins HA, MacKenzie MR, Fudenberg HH. Hemostatic defects in dysproteinemias. Blood 1970;35(5):695–707.

57. Crash trial collaborators, Shakur H, Roberts I, et al. Effects of tranexamic acid on death, vascular occlusive events, and blood transfusion in trauma patients with significant haemorrhage (CRASH-2): a randomised, placebo-controlled trial. Lancet 2010;376(9734):23–32.

58. Perel P, Ker K, Morales Uribe CH, et al. Tranexamic acid for reducing mortality in emergency and urgent surgery. Cochrane Database Syst Rev 2013;(1):CD010245.

59. Shpilberg O, Blumenthal R, Sofer O, et al. A controlled trial of tranexamic acid therapy for the reduction of bleeding during treatment of acute myeloid leukemia. Leuk Lymphoma 1995;19(1–2):141–4.

60. Wardrop D, Estcourt LJ, Brunskill SJ, et al. Antifibrinolytics (lysine analogues) for the prevention of bleeding in patients with haematological disorders. Cochrane Database Syst Rev 2013;(7):CD009733.

61. ISRCTN 73545489, Trial to evaluate tranexamic acid therapy in thrombocytopenia. Avaialable at: http://www.isrctn.com/ISRCTN73545489. Accessed August 3, 2015.

62. Solomon J, Bofenkamp T, Fahey JL, et al. Platelet prophylaxis in acute non-lymphoblastic leukemia. Lancet 1978;1(8058):267.

63. Sintnicolaas K, Velden K, Sizoo W, et al. Comparison of prophylactic and therapeutic single-donor platelet transfusions in patients with acute leukaemia. Br J Haematol 1982;50:684.

64. Steffens I, Harrison JF, Taylor CPF. A dose response study of platelet transfusion: comparison between triple dose apheresis platelet transfusion and three split standard transfusions. Haematologica 2002;87(Suppl 1).

65. WHO. WHO handbook for reporting results of cancer treatment, vol. 48. Geneva (Switzerland): World Health Organisation; 1979.

66. Ajani JA, Welch SR, Raber MN, et al. Comprehensive criteria for assessing therapy-induced toxicity. Cancer Invest 1990;8(2):147–59.

Assessing the Rationale and Effectiveness of Frozen Plasma Transfusions

An Evidence-based Review

Alan Tinmouth, MD, MSc, FRCPC[a,b,c],*

KEYWORDS

- Frozen plasma • Hemostasis • Bleeding • Prophylaxis • Appropriateness

KEY POINTS

- The primary indications for frozen plasma transfusions are the treatment and prevention of bleeding in patients with prolonged coagulation tests, but there is a lack of well-conducted clinical studies to determine the appropriate indications.
- Most patients with mild coagulation test abnormalities do not have a significant hemostatic defect and do not benefit from frozen plasma transfusions.
- No clinical studies have shown a benefit from prophylactic frozen plasma transfusions to nonbleeding patients or before invasive procedures.
- Early transfusion of frozen plasma in massive transfusions is important but current evidence does not support the use of fixed frozen plasma to red transfusion ratios.
- Inappropriate transfusion of frozen plasma is common and may result in adverse events.

Frozen plasma (FP) is a commonly used blood product. The primary indications for FP transfusions are reversal of coagulopathy and replacement fluid in plasma exchange. In the United States, more than 4 million units of FP are transfused annually.[1] In general, the evidence to support the use of FP is limited,[2–4] which has resulted in significant overuse of the product. This overuse likely results in increased adverse

---

Disclosures: A. Tinmouth is supported by a research award from the Department of Medicine, The Ottawa Hospital and is a medical consultant to the Canadian Blood Services. The research for this article was partially supported by grants from the Canadian Institutes of Research and the Canadian Blood Services (86459 and 102538).

a Department of Medicine, Ottawa Hospital, University of Ottawa, 501 Smyth Road, Ottawa, Ontario K1H 8L6, Canada; b Department of Pathology and Laboratory Medicine, Ottawa Hospital, University of Ottawa, 501 Smyth Road, Ottawa, Ontario K1H 8L6, Canada; c Clinical Epidemiology Program, University of Ottawa Centre for Transfusion Research, Ottawa Health Research Institute, 501 Smyth Road, Ottawa, Ontario K1H 8L6, Canada
* 501 Smyth Road, Ottawa, Ontario K1H 8L6, Canada.
E-mail address: atinmouth@ohri.ca

Hematol Oncol Clin N Am 30 (2016) 561–572
http://dx.doi.org/10.1016/j.hoc.2016.01.003
0889-8588/16/$ – see front matter © 2016 Elsevier Inc. All rights reserved.

complications of FP. This article reviews the rationale for the use of FP and the evidence supporting the use and effectiveness of FP transfusions.

FROZEN PLASMA PRODUCTS

Plasma is collected as part of whole blood collections with subsequent separation by centrifugation or by apheresis technology. Within 8 hours of collection, plasma is designated as fresh FP (FFP). Most apheresis plasma is still FFP, but, currently, plasma from whole blood collection is most commonly frozen within 24 hours and referred to as FP-24. In addition, the demand for rapidly available plasma for patients with trauma has resulted in thawed FP being stored for up to 5 days before use. The levels of factor V and VIII decline during longer prestorage holds and after thawing, but adequate levels of all factors are maintained.[5,6] As a result, FFP, FP-24, and thawed plasma are largely used interchangeably in clinical practice. This article uses the term FP generically to refer to all plasma products unless specifically indicated.

More recently, virally inactivated plasma, either individual plasma units (methylene blue, amotosalen–ultraviolet A (UVA), riboflavin-UVA), or pooled solvent-detergent-treated plasma have become available. Laboratory studies show small differences in coagulation or inhibitory proteins in the various pathogen inactivated plasma products,[7–11] but the clinical studies performed to date have not shown any differences in clinical efficacy.[12–15]

RATIONALE FOR FROZEN PLASMA USE

A simple paradigm for the use of FP to treat or prevent bleeding has been described[16,17]: (1) abnormal coagulation tests represent a decrease in levels of coagulation factors that could contribute to bleeding; (2) FP transfusions increase the levels of coagulation factors and correct the coagulation test abnormalities; (3) the correction of the coagulation test abnormality decreases bleeding (**Fig. 1**). However, there are important limitations to each of these 3 tenets.

A prolonged or abnormal coagulation test may not reflect a clinically significant reduction in the coagulation factor levels. Decreases in coagulation factor levels prolong either the activated partial thromboplastin time (aPTT) and/or the prothrombin time, commonly reported as the International Normalized Ratio (INR), but the risk of

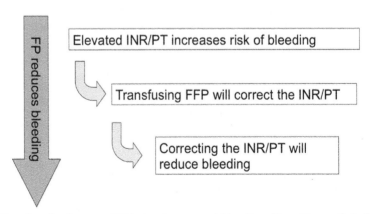

Fig. 1. Paradigm for the use of FP to treat or prevent bleeding. (*From* Tinmouth A. Evidence for a rationale use of frozen plasma for the treatment and prevention of bleeding. Transfus Apher Sci 2012;46(3):294; with permission.)

bleeding only increases when the coagulation levels decrease below a minimum he- mostatic threshold (30% for most factors).[17,18] For the INR, the coagulation factor levels do not decrease below the minimum hemostatic threshold until the INR is greater than 1.7[18] (**Fig. 2**). The lack of correlation between abnormal coagulations and increased bleeding risk was shown in a systematic review of 25 studies (1 ran- domized controlled trial and 24 observational studies) that showed no increase in bleeding associated with prolonged coagulation tests.[16]

FP transfusions increase the levels of the coagulation factors, but the effect on the INR and aPTT depends on the amount of FP transfused and the starting level of the coagulation factors. If the coagulation levels are very low (less than 10%), this results in a significant improvement in the INR or aPTT, but if the initial levels are only mildly decreased then the same increase in coagulation factor levels pro- duces little change in the INR or the aPTT. This lack of efficacy of FP to correct the INR or aPTT in patients with mild coagulation test abnormalities has been repeat- edly shown.[19–24]

Despite routine use of FP transfusions, there are limited data from clinical studies to show that changes in the INR or aPTT are associated with reduced blood loss. A recently updated systematic review found no evidence of decreased bleeding from either therapeutic or prophylactic FP transfusions in 80 randomized controlled trials.[2,3] This systematic review found a more rapid correction of warfarin-induced coagulop- athy with prothrombin complex concentrates (PCCs) compared with FP but no differ- ence in clinical outcomes. A more rapid correction and complete correction of warfarin-related coagulopathy with PCCs has been shown in prospective randomized controlled trials,[25–28] but these prospective studies did not result in reduced red cell transfusion requirements or mortality compared with FP.[29]

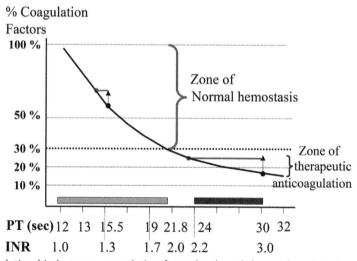

Fig. 2. Relationship between coagulation factor levels and the prothrombin time (PT) and INR. Coagulation factor levels equal to or greater than 30% are sufficient for hemostasis. As indicated by the 2 vertical arrows, the increase in coagulation factors from a fixed dose of FP results in smaller or larger changes in the INR. (*From* Callum J, Dzik WH. The use of blood components prior to invasive bedside procedures: a critical appraisal. In: Mintz PD, editor. Transfusion therapy: clinical principles and practice, 3. Bethesda (MD): AABB Press; 2010. p. 3; with permission.)

INDICATIONS FOR FROZEN PLASMA TRANSFUSIONS

Recommendations for the transfusion of FP, as reflected in national guidelines for the use of FP,[30–33] have remained consistent over the years (**Box 1**).[34] However, the clinical evidence to support these recommendations is limited. The following section examines the evidence for the use of FP in more specific clinical settings.

Prophylactic Frozen Plasma Transfusions for Nonbleeding Patients, and Before Invasive Procedures

FP transfusions are frequently given to patients before invasive procedures or surgery, or to prevent bleeding in patients at higher risk of bleeding. From observational studies, prophylactic use of FP accounts for 24% to 48% of all FP transfusions.[35–37]

The prophylactic use of FP to reduce bleeding has never been shown to reduce bleeding.[2,3] No difference in the rates of intraventricular hemorrhage was seen in 776 neonates randomized to receive FP or volume expanders.[38] Similarly, no differences in bleeding outcomes were seen in 276 patients with acute pancreatitis who were randomly allocated to receive FP or a colloid solution.[39]

More commonly, prophylactic FP is transfused before nonsurgical invasive procedures. A limited number of prospective studies have evaluated the use of FP in these settings. However, the risk of bleeding with these procedures is low even in patients with abnormal coagulation tests who do not receive FP transfusions. A systematic review showed no increase in bleeding risk following bedside invasive procedures in patients with abnormal coagulation tests compared with patients with normal coagulation tests.[16]

More recently, 2 small randomized controlled trials evaluated the use of FP transfusions before invasive procedures. The first study randomized 72 ICU patients requiring a tracheostomy who had mild coagulation abnormalities to receive hemostatic transfusions (FP and/or platelet transfusions) to correct the coagulopathy or to receive no treatment.[40] The amount of blood loss was equal in the transfused and nontransfused groups, and the proportion of the patients with either mild bleeding (51% vs 66%, $P = .16$) or major bleeding (5% vs 9%, $P = .67$) was similar. The second study randomized 81 ICU patients with an INR between 1.5 and 3.0 to receive an FP transfusion or

---

Box 1
Generally accepted indications for FP transfusions

1. Active bleeding, or before surgery or an invasive procedure in patients (adults and neonates) with acquired deficiencies of 1 or more coagulation factors as shown by an increased INR, prothrombin time, or aPTT, when no alternative therapies are available or appropriate

2. Immediate correction of vitamin K deficiency or reversal of warfarin effect in patient with active bleeding, or before surgery or an invasive procedure (in conjunction with the use of Vitamin K)

3. Disseminated intravascular coagulation or consumptive coagulopathy with active bleeding

4. Thrombotic thrombocytopenic purpura

5. Active bleeding, or before surgery or an invasive procedure in patients with a congenital factor deficiency when no alternative therapies are available or appropriate

Adapted from Stanworth SJ, Tinmouth AT. Plasma transfusion and use of albumin. In: Simon TL, Snyder EL, Stowell CP, et al, editors. Rossi's principles of transfusion medicine. Wiley-Blackwell; 2009; with permission.

no transfusion before invasive procedures.[41] No differences in bleeding between the two groups were observed but the study did not have sufficient power to evaluate the planned end point of noninferiority for major bleeding.[42] An additional study evaluating to use of FP compared with PCC before surgery or invasive procedures found no difference in hemostatic efficacy in the subgroup of 28 patients undergoing invasive procedures.[28]

Overall, there is a lack of evidence to guide prophylactic FP transfusions. There is no evidence to support transfusing FP in the absence of bleeding to correct a coagulopathy. The low risk of bleeding associated with nonsurgical invasive procedures and the lack of benefit in small randomized controlled trials argue against routine prophylactic transfusion of FP. The upper limit of the INR for not transfusing FP before invasive procedures is not known but many centers have increased the threshold INR to 1.8 or 2.0. Larger clinical trials evaluating the use of FP before nonsurgical invasive procedures are required to provide definitive evidence regarding the INR threshold for FP before invasive procedures and to help change current practice.

Cardiac Surgery

Epidemiologic transfusion studies suggest that cardiac surgery represents 13% to 19% of all FP use.[36,37] However, the proportion of patients transfused with FP varies widely between centers and these differences in transfusion rates are unlikely to be explained by differences in patient populations.[34] In the setting of cardiac surgery, FP may be given intraoperatively or postoperatively for bleeding, or postoperatively to prevent bleeding in patients with abnormal coagulation tests. A recent systematic review identified 14 trials (700 cardiac surgery patients) comparing prophylactic FFP with no FFP.[43] Patients receiving FP had greater reduction in the prothrombin time (mean difference, −0.71; 95% confidence interval, −1.29, −0.13), but this was not associated with any differences in mortality or blood loss during the first 24 hours. Based on this review, the investigators concluded that there was no evidence to support the prophylactic use of FP in cardiac surgery with no coagulopathy and insufficient evidence in patients with coagulopathy or in bleeding patients.[43]

Liver Disease

Patients with advanced liver disease or cirrhosis frequently have abnormal coagulation tests results, and may be treated with FP before invasive procedures or for bleeding. This finding may represent up to 19% of patients receiving FP.[37] However, the overall hemostatic profile in these patients may not represent an increase in bleeding risk. As recently described, the hemostatic profile of patients with liver disease is complex, with decreases in coagulation factor levels and platelets that is offset by increases in factor VIII and von Willebrand levels and decreases in the inhibitors of coagulation and proteins C and S.[44,45] Recent studies suggest that liver disease represents a balanced hemostatic picture rather than a coagulopathic state.[44–46] Given this understanding, the benefit of FP transfusions in patients with liver disease is unclear. No recent randomized controlled trials have evaluated the use of FP in patients with liver disease. In a recent observational study of 100 patients with liver disease, Youssef and colleagues[22] showed that FP transfusions were often ineffective in correcting coagulation test abnormalities. A similar lack of efficacy for FP transfusions in patients with liver disease has been reported in patients with cirrhosis[20] and patients undergoing liver transplant.[14,15] The lack of efficacy of FP transfusions in patients with liver disease is further supported by studies showing no increase in bleeding following liver biopsy in patients with abnormal coagulation tests.[47] No prospective clinical studies have evaluated the effect of FP transfusions in patients with liver disease who are bleeding. However, there is the potential concern that transfusing FP could either increase the risk of thrombotic potential or exacerbate bleeding by further increasing already increased portal pressures.[48]

Warfarin Reversal

Historically, FP transfusions have been recommended for urgent reversal of warfarin in bleeding patients or patients requiring urgent surgery when there is not sufficient time for vitamin K admiration to have an effect. Clinical studies have shown that vitamin K corrects the INR in 6 to 12 hours when given intravenously.[49,50] Data from retrospective studies showed partial correction of the prothrombin time or INR, but the correction is only partial, with many patients continuing to have an INR greater than normal and even greater than 1.5.[26,29,31] Two recent large randomized controlled trials have compared the effectiveness of FP and a 4-factor PCC in correcting the INR in patients on warfarin who were bleeding,[25] or required surgery or an invasive procedures.[28] In both studies, an adjusted dose of FP was given based on the INR (INR 2 to <4 = 10 mL/kg; INR 4–6 = 12 mL/kg; INR>6 = 15 mL/kg). In the study evaluating bleeding patients, only 9.6% (95% confidence interval, 3.9–15.3) of patients transfused with FP achieved an INR less than 1.3 as measured 0.5 hours after the start of the infusion.[25] In contrast, a significantly higher proportion of patients receiving 4-factor PCC, 62.2% (95% confidence interval, 52.6–71.8), had an INR less than 1.3 at 0.5 hours after infusion. These differences persisted up to 12 hours after transfusion. The hemostatic efficacy of FP, 65.4% (95% confidence interval, 56.2, 74.5), was not significantly different in patients receiving PCC (72.4%; 95% confidence interval, 63.6, 81.3). A subgroup analysis of patients with musculoskeletal or visible bleeding showed decreased hemostatic efficacy with FP transfusions at 4 hours (difference, −32.6; 95% confidence interval, −60.7, −4.5) but not at 24 hours. Because no other clinical data were presented (eg, red cell transfusions or hemoglobin levels), the overall clinical importance of the improved hemostasis observed at 4 hours is not clear.

In the study evaluating FP and PCC before surgery or invasive procedures, similar results were shown.[28] Fewer patients receiving FP had correction of their INR to less than 1.3 immediately following infusion, 8% versus 55% (difference 45·3%; 95% confidence interval, 31·9, 56·4). Patients receiving FP also had reduced hemostasis compared with patients receiving PCC (difference, 14.3%; 95% confidence interval, 2.8–25.8), but there were no differences in red blood cell transfusions between the two groups.

Taken together, these studies[25,28] show that FP corrects the INR in patients on warfarin but the correction is only partial and is less than that achieved with a 4-factor PCC. No studies have evaluated the relative clinical hemostatic efficacy of FP compared with no treatment, but these two recent studies[25,28] suggest that FP could have reduced hemostatic efficacy for the reversal of warfarin compared with PCCs in some settings, such as visible/musculoskeletal bleeds and before surgeries. The more rapid correction of the INR with PCC could also lead to improved clinical outcomes compared with FP in situations of bleeding into critical areas.[24,26] Some retrospective studies have suggested poorer outcomes associated with the use of FP compared with PCCs in patients on warfarin who presented with intracranial hemorrhage,[51] but other studies, including a small prospective randomized controlled trial, have not shown differences in clinical outcomes.[26,52] The relative effectiveness of FP compared with PCC in these patients needs to be determined in larger prospective clinical trials that evaluate both effectiveness and safety.

Trauma/Massive Bleeding

Injury remains a leading cause of death worldwide for younger patients and uncontrolled hemorrhage is a primary cause of death in 40% of these cases. Transfusion therapy is an integral part of supportive treatment of major blood loss. Patients with trauma who present to hospital with major hemorrhage are treated using an integrated approach termed damage-control resuscitation, which focuses on (1) the use of abbreviated surgery and/or interventional radiology to stop bleeding; and (2) best supportive care, including blood and clotting product transfusion. The latter usually includes the use of massive transfusion protocols, which often specify early empiric delivery of FP in a fixed 1:1 ratio with red cells to address the acute coagulopathy of trauma, which increases risks of major hemorrhage and early mortality. Multiple observational studies have suggested improved survival with higher ratio of FP to red cell transfusions; however, these studies have considerable methodologic concerns, most notably survivorship bias (ie, patients who die quickly after arrival at hospital do not survive long enough to get higher doses of FP), which limit any conclusions of the benefit of a 1:1 FP to red cell transfusion ratio.[3,53] More recently, results from the PROPPR trial (Pragmatic, Randomized Optimal Platelet and Plasma Ratios) have been reported.[54] In this randomized controlled trial, higher dose FP transfusion (1:1 ratio with red cells) did not reduce mortality compared with lower dose FP transfusions (1:2 ratio with red cells) (12.7% vs 17.0%; difference, -4.2%; 95% confidence interval, -9.6%, 1.1]). Although early use of FP is likely an important part of the treatment of patients with trauma with hemorrhage, there is not sufficient evidence to determine the optimal transfusion protocols for FP.

Thrombotic Thrombocytopenic Purpura

Based on a randomized controlled trial of 102 patients, which showed improved overall survival with plasma exchange with FP compared with FP infusion,[55] plasma exchange with FP remains the gold standard for treatment.[56,57] Treatment with plasmapheresis and replacement with FP provides a source of the cleaving protein for von Willebrand multimers (ADAMTS13 [A disintegrin and metalloprotease with thrombospondin type 1 motif 13]), and removes both antibodies to ADAMTS13 and ultralarge von Willebrand multimers, which promote the pathologic formation of platelet-rich thrombi. Alternative plasma products such as cryosupernatant plasma and solvent-detergent plasma[58,59] have been shown to be effective as a replacement fluid in plasma exchange for patients with Thrombotic thrombocytopenic purpura (TTP). However, there are no definitive randomized studies that define either the optimal type of plasma (FP, cryosupernatant, or solvent-detergent–treated FP) or the optimal schedule for therapeutic apheresis in patients with TTP.[60]

DOSE OF FROZEN PLASMA

There are important questions about the optimal dose of FP. Given an average concentration of 1 unit/mL for individual coagulation factor levels in FP, transfusing 12 mL/kg (approximately 800–1000 mL) to a 70-kg patient with a 5-L blood volume would be expected to increase levels by approximately 16%. A dose of 10 to 15 mL/kg, which is commonly recommended in guidelines, should be sufficient to increase coagulation factor levels above the hemostatic threshold of 30% for most patients with abnormal coagulation test abnormalities. The optimal dose of FP for clinical use has not been validated or defined in larger trials. In practice, larger doses of FP up to 20 mL/kg may be required to correct the INR or aPTT,[61] particularly in patients with prolonged coagulation tests or specific conditions such as disseminated intravascular coagulation, critical illnesses,[61] or liver disease.[22] However, the clinical benefit of transfusing higher doses of FP is not known, and there may be an increased risk of adverse effects, particularly related to circulatory overload.[62]

SUMMARY

FP is routinely used to correct abnormal coagulation results with the goal of stopping or preventing bleeding. However, repeated audits of FP use continue to show inappropriate rates of 30% or higher.[60,63–66] Although there is a paucity of good clinical evidence to define the appropriate use of FP transfusions, there is reasonable evidence, both indirect and direct, to determine the situations in which there is little clinical benefit from FP transfusions. The 2 largest reasons for inappropriate use are an INR less than or equal to 1.5 and the transfusion of FP in the absence of bleeding.[33,34] A recent audit of UK FP transfusion showed similar results: 12% of all FP transfusions were given in the absence of bleeding or a planned procedure and 20% of patients had an INR less than or equal to 1.5[33] There have been no clinical trials that have shown the effectiveness of prophylactic transfusions of FP, which represents up to 50% of the use of this product.[37,38] In addition, there is no evidence that abnormal coagulation tests are associated with increased bleeding, and transfusing FP has little effect in correcting mild to moderate increases in the INR. Simply recognizing this evidence is important in reducing the inappropriate use of FP and avoiding unnecessary adverse transfusion reactions. Further research is needed to help to delineate the appropriate indications and dosing for FP transfusions, especially compared with other hemostatic therapies such as PCCs and other factor concentrates.

REFERENCES

1. Report of the US Department of Health and Human Services. The 2009 national blood collection and utilization survey report. Washington, DC: US Department of Health and Human Services; 2011.
2. Stanworth SJ, Brunskill SJ, Hyde CJ, et al. Is fresh frozen plasma clinically effective? a systematic review of randomized controlled trials. Br J Haematol 2004; 126(1):139–52.
3. Yang L, Stanworth S, Hopewell S, et al. Is fresh-frozen plasma clinically effective? An update of a systematic review of randomized controlled trials. Transfusion 2012;52:1673–86.
4. Murad MH, Stubbs JR, Gandhi MJ, et al. The effect of plasma transfusion on morbidity and mortality: a systematic review and meta-analysis. Transfusion 2010;50:1370–83.
5. Sheffield WP, Bhakta V, Jenkins C, et al. Conversion to the buffy coat method and quality of frozen plasma derived from whole blood donations in Canada. Transfusion 2010;50(5):1043–9.
6. Sheffield WP, Bhakta V, Mastronardi C, et al. Changes in coagulation factor activity and content of di(2-ethylhexyl)phthalate in frozen plasma units during refrigerated storage for up to five days after thawing. Transfusion 2012;52(3):493–502.
7. Irsch J, Pinkoski L, Corash L, et al. INTERCEPT plasma: comparability with conventional fresh-frozen plasma based on coagulation function–an in vitro analysis. Vox Sang 2010;98(1):47–55.
8. Osselaer JC, Debry C, Goffaux M, et al. Coagulation function in fresh-frozen plasma prepared with two photochemical treatment methods: methylene blue and amotosalen. Transfusion 2008;48(1):108–17.

9. Schlenke P, Hervig T, Isola H, et al. Photochemical treatment of plasma with amotosalen and UVA light: process validation in three European blood centers. Transfusion 2008;48(4):697–705.

10. Garwood M, Cardigan RA, Drummond O, et al. The effect of methylene blue photoinactivation and methylene blue removal on the quality of fresh-frozen plasma. Transfusion 2003;43:1238–47.

11. Sheffield WP, Bhakta V, Talbot K, et al. Quality of frozen transfusable plasma prepared from whole blood donations in Canada: an update. Transfus Apher Sci 2013;49(3):440–6.

12. Bartelmaos T, Chabanel A, Léger J, et al. Plasma transfusion in liver transplantation: a randomized, double-blind, multicenter clinical comparison of three virally secured plasma. Transfusion 2013;53(6):1335–45.

13. Bindi ML, Miccoli M, Marietta M, et al. Solvent detergent vs. fresh frozen plasma in cirrhotic patients undergoing liver transplant surgery: a prospective randomized control study. Vox Sang 2013;105(2):137–43.

14. Williamson LM, Llewelyn CA, Fisher NC, et al. A randomized trial of solvent/detergent-treated and standard fresh-frozen plasma in the coagulopathy of liver disease and liver transplantation. Transfusion 1999;39(11–12):1227–34.

15. Mintz PD, Bass NM, Petz LD, et al. Photochemically treated fresh frozen plasma for transfusion of patients with acquired coagulopathy of liver disease. Blood 2006;107(9):3753–60.

16. Segal JB, Dzik WH. Paucity of studies to support that abnormal coagulation test results predict bleeding in the setting of invasive procedures: an evidence-based review. Transfusion 2005;45(9):1413–25.

17. Tinmouth A. Evidence for a rationale use of frozen plasma for the treatment and prevention of bleeding. Transfus Apher Sci 2012;46(3):293–8.

18. Callum J, Dzik WH. The use of blood components prior to invasive bedside procedures: a critical appraisal. In: Mintz PD, editor. Transfusion therapy: clinical principles and practice, 3. Bethesda (MD): AABB Press; 2010. p. 1–36.

19. Holland LL, Brooks JP. Toward rational fresh frozen plasma transfusion: the effect of plasma transfusion on coagulation test results. Am J Clin Pathol 2006;126(1):133–9.

20. Abdel-Wahab OI, Healy B, Dzik WH. Effect of fresh-frozen plasma transfusion on prothrombin time and bleeding in patients with mild coagulation abnormalities. Transfusion 2006;46(8):1279–85.

21. Makris M, Greaves M, Phillips WS, et al. Emergency oral anticoagulant reversal: the relative efficacy of infusions of fresh frozen plasma and clotting factor concentrate on correction of the coagulopathy. Thromb Haemost 1997;77(3):477–80.

22. Youssef WI, Salazar F, Dasarathy S, et al. Role of fresh frozen plasma infusion in correction of coagulopathy of chronic liver disease: a dual phase study. Am J Gastroenterol 2003;98(6):1391–4.

23. Gazzard BG, Henderson JM, Williams R. The use of fresh frozen plasma or a concentrate of factor IX as replacement therapy before liver biopsy. Gut 1975;16(8):621–5.

24. Fredriksson K, Norrving B, Stromblad LG. Emergency reversal of anticoagulation after intracerebral hemorrhage. Stroke 1992;23(7):972–7.

25. Sarode R, Milling TJ Jr, Refaai MA, et al. Efficacy and safety of a 4-factor prothrombin complex concentrate in patients on vitamin K antagonists presenting with major bleeding: a randomized, plasma-controlled, phase IIIb study. Circulation 2013;128(11):1234–43.

26. Boulis NM, Bobek MP, Schmaier A, et al. Use of factor IX complex in warfarin-related intracranial hemorrhage. Neurosurgery 1999;45(5):1113–8.

27. Demeyere R, Gillardin S, Arnout J, et al. Comparison of fresh frozen plasma and prothrombin complex concentrate for the reversal of oral anticoagulants in patients undergoing cardiopulmonary bypass surgery: a randomized study. Vox Sang 2010;99(3):251–60.

28. Goldstein JN, Refaai MA, Milling TJ Jr, et al. Four-factor prothrombin complex concentrate versus plasma for rapid vitamin K antagonist reversal in patients needing urgent surgical or invasive interventions: a phase 3b, open-label, non-inferiority, randomised trial. Lancet 2015;385(9982):2077–87.

29. Johansen M, Wikkelsø A, Lunde J, et al. Prothrombin complex concentrate for reversal of vitamin K antagonist treatment in bleeding and non-bleeding patients. Cochrane Database Syst Rev 2015;(7):CD010555.

30. O'Shaughnessy DF, Atterbury C, Bolton Maggs P, et al. British Committee for Standards in Haematology, Blood Transfusion Task Force. Guidelines for the use of fresh-frozen plasma, cryoprecipitate and cryosupernatant. Br J Haematol 2004;126(1):11–28.

31. American Society of Anesthesiologists Task Force on Perioperative Blood Management. Practice guidelines for perioperative blood management: an updated report by the American Society of Anesthesiologists Task Force on Perioperative Blood Management. Anesthesiology 2015;122(2):241–75.

32. Canadian Medical Association Expert Working Group. Guidelines for red blood cell and plasma transfusion for adults and children. Can Med Assoc J 1997; 156(11 suppl):S1–24.

33. Lundberg GD. Practice parameter for the use of fresh-frozen plasma, cryoprecipitate, and platelets. Fresh-Frozen plasma, cryoprecipitate, and platelets administration practice guidelines development task force of the College of American Pathologists. JAMA 1994;271:777–81.

34. Stanworth SJ, Tinmouth AT. Plasma transfusion and use of albumin. In: Simon TL, Snyder EL, Stowell CP, et al, editors. Rossi's principles of transfusion medicine. Oxford (UK): Wiley-Blackwell; 2009. p. 287–9.

35. Dzik W, Rao A. Why do physicians request fresh frozen plasma? Transfusion 2004;44:1393–4.

36. Stanworth SJ, Grant-Casey J, Lowe D, et al. The use of fresh-frozen plasma in England: high levels of inappropriate use in adults and children. Transfusion 2011; 51:62–70.

37. Tinmouth A, Fergusson DA, McIntyre L, et al. High rates of inappropriate frozen plasma utilization based on expert medical rating; results of a multicentre Canadian study. Transfusion 2012;52(3S):115A.

38. A randomized trial comparing the effect of prophylactic intravenous fresh frozen plasma, gelatin or glucose on early mortality and morbidity in preterm babies. The Northern Neonatal Nursing Initiative [NNNI] Trial Group. Eur J Pediatr 1996;155(7):580–8.

39. Leese T, Holliday M, Watkins M, et al. A multicentre controlled clinical trial of high-volume fresh frozen plasma therapy in prognostically severe acute pancreatitis. Ann R Coll Surg Engl 1991;73(4):207–14.

40. Veelo DP, Vlaar AP, Dongelmans DA, et al. Correction of subclinical coagulation disorders before percutaneous dilatational tracheotomy. Blood Transfus 2012;10: 213–20.

41. Muller MC, de Jonge E, Arbous MS, et al. Transfusion of fresh frozen plasma in non-bleeding ICU patients–TOPIC trial: study protocol for a randomized controlled trial. Trials 2011;12:266.
42. Müller MC, Arbous MS, Spoelstra-de Man AM, et al. Transfusion of fresh-frozen plasma in critically ill patients with a coagulopathy before invasive procedures: a randomized clinical trial (CME). Transfusion 2015;55(1):26–35.
43. Desborough M, Sandu R, Brunskill SJ, et al. Fresh frozen plasma for cardiovascular surgery. Cochrane Database Syst Rev 2015;(7):CD007614.
44. Tripodi A, Mannucci PM. The coagulopathy of chronic liver disease. N Engl J Med 2011;365(2):147–56.
45. Lisman T, Porte RJ. Rebalanced hemostasis in patients with liver disease: evidence and clinical consequences. Blood 2010;116(6):878–85.
46. Tripodi A, Salerno F, Chantarangkul V, et al. Evidence of normal thrombin generation in cirrhosis despite abnormal conventional coagulation tests. Hepatology 2005;41:553–8.
47. McVay PA, Toy PTCY. Lack of increased bleeding after liver biopsy in patients with mild hemostatic abnormalities. Am J Clin Pathol 1990;94:747–53.
48. Garcia-Tsao G, Groszmann RJ, Fisher RL, et al. Portal pressure, presence of gastroesophageal varices and variceal bleeding. Hepatology 1985;5(3):419–24.
49. Watson HG, Baglin T, Laidlaw SL, et al. A comparison of the efficacy and rate of response to oral and intravenous vitamin K in reversal of over-anticoagulation with warfarin. Br J Haematol 2001;115(1):145–9.
50. Lubetsky A, Yonath H, Olchovsky D, et al. Comparison of oral vs intravenous phytonadione (vitamin K1) in patients with excessive anticoagulation: a prospective randomized controlled study. Arch Intern Med 2003;163(20):2469–73.
51. Frontera JA, Gordon E, Zach V, et al. Reversal of coagulopathy using prothrombin complex concentrates is associated with improved outcome compared to fresh frozen plasma in warfarin-associated intracranial hemorrhage. Neurocrit Care 2014;21(3):397–406.
52. Parry-Jones AR, Di Napoli M, Goldstein JN, et al. Reversal strategies for vitamin K antagonists in acute intracerebral hemorrhage. Ann Neurol 2015;78(1):54–62.
53. Rajasekhar A, Gowing R, Zarychanski R, et al. Survival of trauma patients after massive red blood cell transfusion using a high or low red blood cell to plasma transfusion ratio. Crit Care Med 2011;39(6):1507–13.
54. Holcomb JB, Tilley BC, Baraniuk S, et al. Transfusion of plasma, platelets, and red blood cells in a 1:1:1 vs a 1:1:2 ratio and mortality in patients with severe trauma: the PROPPR randomized clinical trial. JAMA 2015;313(5):471–82.
55. Rock GA, Shumak KH, Buskard NA. Comparison of plasma exchange with plasma infusion in the treatment of thrombotic thrombocytopenic purpura. Canadian Apheresis Study Group. N Engl J Med 1991;325:393–7.
56. Michael M, Elliott EJ, Ridley GF, et al. Interventions for haemolytic uraemic syndrome and thrombotic thrombocytopenic purpura. Cochrane Database Syst Rev 2009;(1):CD003595.
57. Scully M, Hunt BJ, Benjamin S, et al, British Committee for Standards in Haematology. Guidelines on the diagnosis and management of thrombotic thrombocytopenic purpura and other thrombotic microangiopathies. Br J Haematol 2012; 158(3):323–35.
58. Mintz PD, Neff A, MacKenzie M, et al. A randomized, controlled phase III trial of therapeutic plasma exchange with fresh-frozen plasma (FFP) prepared with amotosalen and ultraviolet A light compared to untreated FFP in thrombotic thrombocytopenic purpura. Transfusion 2006;46(10):1693–704.

59. Scully M, Longair I, Flynn M, et al. Cryosupernatant and solvent detergent fresh-frozen plasma (Octaplas) usage at a single centre in acute thrombotic thrombocytopenic purpura. Vox Sang 2007;93(2):154–8.

60. Arnold DM, Lauzier F, Whittingham H, et al. A multifaceted strategy to reduce inappropriate use of frozen plasma transfusions in the intensive care unit. J Crit Care 2011;26(6):636.e7–13.

61. Chowdary P, Saayman AG, Paulus U, et al. Efficacy of standard dose and 30 ml/kg fresh frozen plasma in correcting laboratory parameters of haemostasis in critically ill patients. Br J Haematol 2004;125(1):69–73.

62. Andrezejewski C, Popovsky MA. Transfusion-associated adverse pulmonary sequelae: widening our perspective. Transfusion 2005;45:1048–50.

63. Hui CH, Williams I, Davis K. Clinical audit of the use of fresh-frozen plasma and platelets in a tertiary teaching hospital and the impact of a new transfusion request form. Intern Med J 2005;35(5):283–8.

64. Yeh CJ, Wu CF, Hsu WT, et al. Transfusion audit of fresh-frozen plasma in southern Taiwan. Vox Sang 2006;91(3):270–4.

65. Pybus S, MacCormac A, Houghton A, et al. Inappropriateness of fresh frozen plasma for abnormal coagulation tests. J R Coll Physicians Edinb 2012;42(4):294–300.

66. Tinmouth A, Thompson T, Arnold DM, et al. Utilization of frozen plasma in Ontario: a provincewide audit reveals a high rate of inappropriate transfusions. Transfusion 2013;53(10):2222–9.

Autologous Stem Cell Mobilization and Collection

Yen-Michael S. Hsu, MD, PhD[a],*, Melissa M. Cushing, MD[b],*

KEYWORDS

- G-CSF • Plerixafor • Mobilization • Collection • Transplantation • Stem cell
- Hematopoiesis • Laboratory

KEY POINTS

- The clinical use of mobilization agents is effective to achieve peripheral collection of stem cells.
- Stem cell sources, mobilization strategies, and collection methods may impact graft quality and transplantation outcomes.
- Monitoring and predicting mobilization are critical to coordinate between the various clinical services involved in stem cell transplantation.
- Apheresis-based peripheral blood stem cell collection is safe but requires many periprocedural preparations.

INTRODUCTION

Autologous stem cell transplant can be a curative therapy to restore normal hematopoiesis after myeloablative treatments in patients with lymphocytic malignancies, such as multiple myeloma (MM), non-Hodgkin lymphoma (NHL), Hodgkin lymphoma, and other malignancies. Mobilized hematopoietic stem/progenitor cells (HSPCs) collected by apheresis are the predominant source of stem cells for autologous and allogeneic transplant because of their higher yield and the decreased procedural risk compared with bone marrow (BM) harvest. Patients who have had many cycles of high-dose chemotherapy and/or radiation may have a significantly reduced BM reserve and a poor autologous yield after attempted stem cell mobilization and collection. Owing to the toxicity of prolonged chemotherapy exposure, alternative mobilization agents, and algorithms have been explored continuously for improvement.

[a] Pathology and Laboratory Medicine, Transfusion Medicine and Cellular Therapy, Weill Cornell Medical College, 525 East 68th Street, Box 251, New York, NY 10065, USA; [b] Transfusion Medicine and Cellular Therapy, Weill Cornell Medical College, 525 East 68th Street, Box 251, M09, New York, NY 10065, USA
* Corresponding authors.
E-mail addresses: ysh9001@med.cornell.edu; mec2013@med.cornell.edu

Hematol Oncol Clin N Am 30 (2016) 573–589
http://dx.doi.org/10.1016/j.hoc.2016.01.004
0889-8588/16/$ – see front matter © 2016 Elsevier Inc. All rights reserved.

The clinical practice of HSPC mobilization and collection requires real-time and frequent communication between the clinical transplant team, the apheresis service, and the cellular therapy/stem cell laboratory. These optimized interactions are essential to the success of graft collection for patients who await hematopoietic rescue. There have been several published review articles addressing various aspects of HSPC mobilization. However, very few integrate solutions to the logistical and communication issues between the different services that allow for optimal patient management.

In this article, we review the safety, efficacy, and cost, as well as recent improvements in HSPC mobilization and collection. Finally, we address some of the practical concerns during the coordination of care between the clinical transplant team, the apheresis service and the cellular therapy laboratory. Although the practice continues to evolve, HSPC mobilization for allogeneic donors tends to have less mobilization failure given the allogeneic donor's healthier status and BM reserve compared with diseased autologous donors. There have been several reviews published on the topic of allogeneic mobilization,[1,2] and this review focuses on adult autologous donors, with an occasional reference to allogeneic donors when appropriate.

DISCOVERY OF THE HEMATOPOIETIC STEM CELL NICHE AND CLINICAL TRANSLATION

Since hematopoietic transplantation was established in the 1960s, the intricate cellular mechanisms and interactions of HSPCs and their BM microenvironment or "niche" have been investigated extensively.[3] Studies have shown that the BM niche plays an essential role in determining the ultimate fate of the HSPCs, including cellular trafficking, differentiation, and self-renewal. The main cell types comprising the niche are mesenchymal stem cells, osteoblasts, perivascular stromal cells, and endothelial cells. Various ligands expressed on the surface of or secreted from the niche cells dynamically interact with their cognate receptors on the HSPCs. This highly organized, direct cellular engagement is mediated by a sophisticated lipid raft formation that permits the proximity of signaling molecules to transduce intracellular signals (**Fig. 1**).[4,5] The formation and disassembly of the lipid raft result in HSPC BM retention and mobilization, respectively. Molecular analyses of these interactions have translated into the rapid development of drugs that are used clinically to mobilize BM HSPCs into peripheral circulation, which allows collections by apheresis.

CLINICAL HEMATOPOIETIC STEM/PROGENITOR CELL MOBILIZATION

Quiescent repopulating HSPCs are often tethered to osteoblasts, other stromal cells, and the extracellular matrix in the stem cell niche through a variety of adhesive molecule interactions. Disruption of niche interactions using cytotoxic agents, hematopoietic growth factors, small-molecule chemokine analogs, or even recombinant monoclonal antibodies can lead to release of HSPCs from the BM into the PB.[6] In 2010, Sheppard and colleagues[7] published a systematic review on 28 published randomized, controlled trials evaluating HSPC mobilization/collection strategies. The consensus was that mobilization improvement often comes with increased toxicity; therefore, the selection of a mobilization regimen should be considered and determined based on clinical resources and patient-specific factors. Since 2010, additional published algorithms have addressed some of those considerations (**Table 1**).[8–14]

Chemotherapy Mobilization

It was discovered in the early 1990s that HSPC concentration increased 5- to 15-fold during the postcyclophosphamide (CY) recovery period and that the increase is

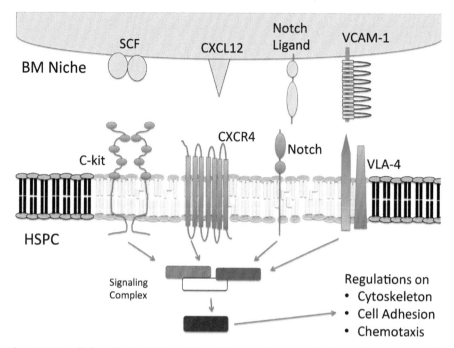

Fig. 1. Intercellular physical interactions between hematopoietic stem/progenitor cells (HSPCs) and BM stromal cells. Several paired receptor–ligand molecules were identified that can physically tether HSPCs to the BM stromal niche cells. Upon activation, C-kit (also known as CD117 or stem cell factor receptor), C-X-C motif receptor 4 (CXCR4), Notch, and very late antigen 4 (VLA-4) are the critical transmembrane HSPC proteins that mediate various intracellular signaling and cellular processes, including cellular migration, morphologic change, adhesion, and cellular quiescence. Lipid raft, shown as the yellow-colored lipid bilayer region on the HSPC cell membrane, was observed to contain a higher concentration of these receptors and their downstream protein complex assemblies. CXCL12, C-X-C motif chemokine ligand 12 or stromal-derived factor 1 (SDF-1); HSPCs, hematopoietic stem and progenitor cells; VCAM-1, vascular cell adhesion molecule 1.

affected by chemotherapy dosage, longer treatment-free period because prior chemotherapy, and by a higher colony forming unit–granulocyte macrophage level.[15] CY is currently the chemotherapy of choice to mobilize HSPCs in autologous patients. High-dose CY chemotherapy in MM patients showed a significant improvement in clinical outcomes.[16] Although higher CY dosage in combination with granulocyte–colony stimulating factor (G-CSF) results in a higher PB CD34$^+$ concentration, the enhanced mobilization effect plateaus and has more frequent adverse events, such as neutropenic fever, blood transfusion, and longer hospitalization.[17] Owing to the unfavorable toxicity profile, the safety and efficacy of alternative mobilization agents were explored.[18,19]

Colony-Stimulating Factors

There are two hematopoietic growth factors approved by the US Food and Drug Administration (FDA) for the mobilization of stem cells: G-CSF and granulocyte–macrophage colony-stimulating factor (GM-CSF).

Table 1
Examples of algorithms to improve mobilization/collection efficiency and yield

Published Strategies	Intervention Algorithm	Outcomes
Jantunen et al,[8] 2012	Addition of plerixafor when PB CD34 <10/µL and WBC >5000/µL on day 5 (sensitivity 97%; specificity 100%)	Improved success in reaching standard collection goal[a]
Douglas et al,[9] 2012	The use of plerixafor as single mobilization agent in adults with multiple myeloma and dialysis-dependent renal injury	Improved success in reaching standard collection goal[a]
Lefrere et al,[10] 2013	Early monitoring of plerixafor-mobilized PB CD34 (3–5 h after infusion), in donors with prior mobilization failure	Increased leukapheresis eligibility and collection success
Storch et al,[11] 2015	Addition of plerixafor for day 4 PB CD34 <10/µL	Reduced leukapheresis operational burden and faster completion of collection
Gutensohn et al,[12] 2010	Initiation of daily PB CD34 monitoring on day 3 of mobilization to determine optimal leukapheresis timing	Reduced G-CSF administration, number of procedures, cost, and time
Duong et al,[13] 2011	Addition of plerixafor when the first collection yield is <0.7 × 10⁶ CD34⁺ cells/kg body weight	Reduced mobilization/collection failure
Horwitz et al,[14] 2012	Use of plerixafor on day 5 for poor G-CSF mobilizers, determined by day-5 PB CD34 of <7/µL	Improved success in reaching standard collection goal[a]

Abbreviations: G-CSF, granulocyte-colony stimulating factor; PB CD34, peripheral Blood CD34 level.
[a] Standard collection goal: 2 to 5 × 10⁶ CD34⁺ cells/kg body weight.
Data from Refs.[8–14]

Granulocyte-colony stimulating factor (filgrastim)

G-CSF is the first-line treatment for HSPC mobilization and has been shown to reduce neutropenia-related infection and enhance posttransplant myeloid recovery.[20] The exact mechanism of G-CSF based mobilization has been intensively investigated, but is still not fully understood. At the molecular level, G-CSF is thought to indirectly destabilize the HSPCs retention in BM by disrupting the C-X-C motif chemokine ligand 12 (CXCL12)/C-X-C motif receptor 4 (CXCR4) axis and increasing the release of proteolytic enzymes (neutrophil elastase and cathepsin G). It has been proposed that G-CSF disrupts the BM niche by attenuating endosteal osteoblasts, modulating intramedullary macrophages, and disrupting the local CXCL12 gradient. The usual administration of G-CSF for HSPC mobilization is subcutaneous injection of 10 µg kg^{-1} day^{-1} with HSPC collection on day 4 or 5. In the autologous mobilization setting after chemotherapy, the G-CSF is well-tolerated given that these patients are usually pancytopenic at baseline. However, rare severe side effects such as leukostasis and splenic rupture have been reported. An additional concern for G-CSF mobilization in the autologous donor is the contamination of BM tumor cells in the autologous graft product.[21]

Modified filgrastim

Polyethylene glycol-conjugated G-CSF (pegfilgrastim) has captured increasing attention owing to its longer half-life and its ability to achieve a more predictable circulating

CD34 concentration. In the setting of autologous transplantation, it only requires a single dose that is independent of donor weight. Therefore, although pegfilgrastim is more expensive than G-CSF per dose, the appropriate use of pegfilgrastim can be more cost effective than G-CSF.[22] However, a comprehensive cost analysis is still required. A recent metaanalysis concluded that pegfilgrastim mobilization is associated with a significantly shorter time to onset of collection and less required leukapheresis procedures. Filgrastim and pegfilgrastim share a similar toxicity profile, and thus pegfilgrastim could be a convenient alternative to G-CSF for mobilizing HSPC.[23] However, it is currently not approved by the FDA for the purpose of HSPC mobilization.

Lenograstim is a glycosylated form of G-CSF that shows comparable mobilization efficacy with reduced dosage compared with the traditional G-CSF.[24] An additional study showed that pegfilgrastim reduced neutropenic fever to a greater extent than filgrastim and lenograstim.[25] Small comparative randomized controlled trials that examined the potency of HSPC mobilization by filgrastim and lenograstim have demonstrated comparable mobilization efficacy to filgrastim.[26,27]

The efficiency of various forms of G-CSF was directly compared and showed that lenograstim ($10 \, \mu g \, kg^{-1} \, day^{-1}$) had significantly higher CD34$^+$ collection yield than filgrastim or pegfilgrastim.[28] However, additional clinical trials evaluating the potency, efficacy, and safety of lenograstim are still needed. Similar to pegfilgrastim, lenograstim has not yet obtained FDA approval for mobilizing HSPC clinically.

Biosimilar granulocyte-colony stimulating factor

To decrease pricing and foster innovative competition, the FDA has created an expedited licensure pathway for the development of biologics that possess similar potency, efficacy, and safety to a reference-approved biologic. However, these biosimilars are not automatically approved for the claimed indication to the reference product. Since the patent expiration of filgrastim (Neupogen) in 2006, several G-CSF biosimilars known as Ratiograstim/Tevagrastim, Nivestim, Zarxio/Filgrastim-sndz, and Grastofil have entered into clinical trials for the purpose of obtaining approvals from the European Medicine Agency and the FDA. One of the major benefits to using these G-CSF biosimilars is the low cost.

Nivestim, one of the G-CSF biosimilars, has recently shown a mild but significant decrease in the number of leukapheresis procedures for autologous donors. In a cohort of 51 patients, Nivestim-induced mobilization shared a similar toxicity profile to the reference filgrastim arm; however, the Nivestim-mobilized graft was associated with a 2-day delay in platelet engraftment.[29] Several completed clinical trials demonstrate that the G-CSF biosimilars have comparable efficacy and safety for HSPC mobilization in both autologous and allogeneic donors.[30,31] In March 2015, Zarxio became the first G-CSF biosimilar approved by the FDA for the same indications as filgrastim (Neupogen), including mobilization of autologous hematopoietic progenitor cell (HPC) for collection. However, a long-term safety evaluation of the biosimilars is still needed.

Granulocyte-macrophage colony-stimulating factor (sargramostim)

Similar to G-CSF, GM-CSF is a growth factor approved by the FDA to hasten myeloid recovery in patients with treatment-related neutropenia. It was noted that GM-CSF could also mobilize HSPCs into the PB. When directly compared with G-CSF, GM-CSF is less efficacious in mobilizing HSPCs with or without chemotherapy.[32–34] When compared with G-CSF, GM-CSF mobilized grafts lead to slower neutrophil engraftment but faster platelet recovery.[35] GM-CSF could further enhance G-CSF–mediated HSPC mobilization in autologous donors after chemotherapy.[36] However, the synergism is not significantly better than the mobilization by G-CSF alone.[33] Thus, it is considered a salvage mobilization regimen in patients who have failed G-CSF mobilization.

Small Molecule Chemokine Analogs and Monoclonal Antibodies

Plerixafor

Plerixafor (also known as AMD3100) is a small bicyclam molecule that reversibly antagonizes the CXCR4 receptor, leading to disruption of CXCL12-CXCR4–supported HSPC retention.[37,38] Before plerixafor's FDA approval in 2008 as a mobilizing agent, two large phase III randomized controlled trials were conducted by DiPersio and colleagues[39,40] that showed a significant increase in circulating CD34+ cells and the graft collection yield mobilized by plerixafor versus placebo and concurrent G-CSF. In addition, comparable engraftment outcomes and adverse events were observed during these trials in both NHL and MM patient cohorts. Plerixafor is generally well-tolerated with rare severe side effects, such as hypotension, dizziness, and thrombocytopenia. The most commonly observed adverse reactions were diarrhea, nausea, and skin erythema at the injection site.

The use of plerixafor has been shown to be helpful in facilitating mobilization in autologous donors that have had repetitive intense systemic chemotherapy, lenalidomide treatment,[41] or worsening disease.[42] Although plerixafor with G-CSF is superior to and comparably safer than G-CSF alone, Devine and colleagues[43] have examined mobilization potency and transplantation outcomes using a mobilization regimen with plerixafor alone versus G-CSF alone. Although plerixafor alone led to an eight-fold increase in PB CD34 count, 5-day G-CSF mobilization has a significantly greater increase in PB CD34 mobilization (>15-fold increase from baseline). Interestingly, the plerixafor mobilized graft contained a lower CD34 content with more mobilized lymphocytes, but resulted in similar engraftment outcomes compared with the G-CSF mobilized graft.[43] In addition, plerixafor plus G-CSF was recently reported to increase the mobilization of HSPCs with greater repopulating potential (CD34+CD133+CD38−) in autologous donors with MM and NHL.[44,45] These findings collectively support the idea that variable mechanisms for disrupting BM niches could differentially liberate different HSPC populations from their specific niches into the circulation.

Stem cell factor (ancestim)

Stem cell factor (SCF), also known as c-kit ligand, is another hematopoietic growth factor produced by perivascular stromal progenitors and endothelial cells.[46] Similar to CXCL12, SCF also has differential splicing protein variants present as soluble or membrane-bound proteins. Upon binding to its cognate receptor, membrane-bound SCF could further upregulate the expression of the very late antigen-4 adhesion molecule that tethers HSPCs to the BM niche. However, the soluble SCF could differentially inhibit this engagement, resulting in the liberation of HSPCs. Ancestim, the recombinant form of human SCF, when used with G-CSF, increases the CD34+ cell yield in poor mobilizers.[47] The most recent published clinical study in 2011 was led by Lapierre and colleagues,[48] which included more than 500 patients with various hematologic malignancies. The administration of ancestim for mobilization has been shown to lead to a 31% success rate in collecting 2×10^6 CD34 kg^{-1} body weight in patients who previously failed mobilization; however, it is also associated with significant reactions, including allergic reactions owing to mast cell degranulation. Johnsen and colleagues[49] have conducted the first randomized, controlled trial comparing the effect of Ancestim with conventional chemotherapy in conjunction with G-CSF. The study showed that although ancestim reduced chemotherapy toxicity, it was also associated with reduced $CD34^+$ HSPC product yield. Currently, ancestim is only approved in Canada and New Zealand. It is not available in the United States.

Recombinant very late antigen-4 (VLA-4) antagonist
Natalizumab is a recombinant humanized anti-VLA-4 monoclonal antibody approved for Crohn's disease and multiple sclerosis; however, it has also been shown to enhance peripheral HSPC mobilization.[50] No clinical trials have been conducted using this VLA-4 inhibitor antibody for HSPC mobilization.

CLINICAL APPROACHES IN COLLECTING MOBILIZED HEMATOPOIETIC STEM/PROGENITOR CELLS

An apheresis procedure is used to collect HSPCs. Leukapheresis selectively removes the mononuclear buffy coat layer to harvest the HSPCs. The goal of stem cell collection is to achieve maximum efficiency by reaching the goal for $CD34^+$ cells collected in the minimum number of apheresis procedures. Efficient HSPC collection is critical owing to the high cost of each leukapheresis procedure and the risk to patients during the procedure.[51] Several clinical trials have established that a minimum of 2×10^6 $CD34^+$ cells kg^{-1} body weight is needed for successful engraftment. However, for autologous stem cell transplantation, 5 to 10×10^6 $CD34^+$ cells kg^{-1} body weight is desirable for faster engraftment (neutrophil and platelet) and less resource utilization.[52,53] To achieve the ideal collection goal in a cost-balanced manner, many groups have proposed various strategies using laboratory data to optimize collection efficiency.[11] Successful collection algorithms depend on optimized mobilization methods, optimal timing of collection using predictive assays, and an efficient leukapheresis procedure. Although many studies have reported successful improvements in collection efficiency, no randomized controlled trials have directly compared the available algorithms.

Predicting Successful Collection

The first challenge during stem cell collection is to determine the ideal time to collect the patient. Certain donor-related variables may impact the ability to achieve the HSPCs collection goal, such as donor age, previous chemotherapy, mobilization regimen, and platelet count at the time of mobilization. Thus each patient needs to be closely monitored to determine the optimal timing for collection. Generally, three approaches have been taken to determine donor readiness for collection: (1) monitoring the white blood cell (WBC) count, (2) PB CD34 count, or (3) HPC enumeration using a Sysmex hematology analyzer. Over time, many comparative studies have been performed to search for the best parameter to predict the success of reaching the collection goal. With the advancement of technology and establishment of assay standardization, preharvest PB CD34 evaluation seems to be the most consistent predictor for yield and successful collection. In addition, the use of PB CD34 can significantly avoid the cost of unnecessary apheresis procedures and product processing.[12] However, different platforms for determining the optimal time for collection all have advantages and disadvantages (**Table 2**).[8,54–62] In general, the optimal timing of apheresis is generally after 5 days of daily G-CSF administration. $CD34^+$ cells tend to begin to increase in the PB by day 4 with a peak on day 5, and generally tend to decrease after day 5. Thus, optimizing the timing of the procedure is critical. The timing of the collection after chemotherapy mobilization depends on the chemotherapy regimen.

White blood cells
HSPC mobilization is associated with the egress of immune cells into PB. The simple WBC count is an inexpensive laboratory test with a fast turnaround time that can be

Table 2
Commonly used laboratory parameters to predict HSPC mobilization and collection outcomes

Conventional Laboratory Predictors	Advantages	Disadvantages	References
PB CD34	Best predictor for collection yield	May have reduced HSPC yield prediction in MDS/MPD patients	8,54–56,63
	Standardized by ISHAGE protocol	Limited access	
	Good predictor for collection efficiency	Complex testing	
	—	Slow TAT	
Automated HPC analyzer	Better predictor than WBC or MNC for leukapheresis timing	Inferior to PB CD34	57–60
	Better predictor than WBC for predicting PB CD34	Expensive platform	
	Quick TAT	—	
	FDA approved	—	
WBC	Inexpensive test	Inferior to PB CD34 and automated HPC analyzer	8,61,62
	Quick TAT	Variability owing to autologous donor disease status	
	Better predictor ($R^2 = 0.19$) than albumin or hematocrit	—	
	Good (negative) predictor for collection efficiency	—	

Abbreviations: FDA, US Food and Drug Administration; HSPC, hematopoietic stem and progenitor cells; ISHAGE, International Society of Hematotherapy and Graft Engineering; MDS/MPD, myelodysplastic syndrome/myeloproliferative disorder; MNC, mononuclear cells; PB CD34, peripheral blood CD34 level; TAT, turn-around time; WBC, white blood count.
Data from Refs.[8,54–63]

used to determine the optimal timing for HSPC collection.[63,64] In a retrospective study, Verlinden and colleagues[62] proposed peripheral WBC count as a stronger predictor for HSPC collection efficiency than PB CD34 count. However, it should be noted that the study did not use the more accurate International Society of Hematotherapy and Graft Engineering protocol to quantify the CD34 population. In fact, a recent survey have found that only 16 out of 92 surveyed transplant facilities use WBC count as a trigger for HSPC leukapheresis.[65] Other studies showed WBC to be less superior to a direct quantification of PB CD34+ concentration.[54–56] Although the WBC count is viewed overall as an inferior, indirect surrogate compared with PB CD34, depending on the resources and logistic considerations in an institution, it may be very helpful.

Peripheral blood CD34 count
CD34 is a protein that belongs to a family of sialomucins whose function has yet to be defined. However, it has been used for the past 40 years as a surrogate marker for hematopoietic progenitors enriched with repopulating stem cells. Although the use of CD34 analysis by flow cytometry is well-established, it was not standardized until the introduction of the International Society of Hematotherapy and Graft Engineering (ISHAGE) protocol.[66]

Because the quality of the HSPC graft is partially evaluated by its CD34 content, PB CD34 was measured and determined to be a reliable predictor for adequate mobilization. A pre-harvest PB CD34 level can be used to initiate leukapheresis. Several studies have found that PB CD34+ concentration positively correlates with G-CSF dosage in both autologous and healthy allogeneic donors.[67] In addition, PB (preharvest) CD34 correlates well with the final product yield.[68] This predictive correlation also seems to hold with addition of plerixafor, which does not change the strong relationship between the preharvest CD34 and the first product CD34 yield or product collection efficiency.[60,69]

Hematopoietic progenitor cell count

The FDA has approved the use of the HPC count on an automated hematology analyzer (Sysmex, Kobe, Japan) for predicting when to begin apheresis for stem cell collection. The Sysmex analyzer uses the combination of polyoxyethylene nonionic surfactant (to induce red blood cell lysis) and polymethine dye (an immature myeloid stain) to detect and enumerate HPCs, using both optical and general flow cytometry-based detection systems.[70] The HPC number does not correlate well with CD34+ cell count in PB, but because it is known that all HSPCs do not express CD34, it was postulated that HPCs measured by Sysmex include some HSPCs that are CD34 negative. The HPC measurement is rapidly available and less expensive, but it is much more difficult to use to predict optimal timing of apheresis.[60]

Donor-specific factors

Autologous donors often have preexisting hematopoietic abnormalities and their BM HSPC reserve can be variably compromised by prior cytotoxic chemotherapy and radiation exposure. Jantunen and colleagues[71] have tried to predict the mobilization based on the clinical characteristics and failed to discover any significant predictive parameters in an NHL cohort. Interestingly, in a small MM cohort, Duong and colleagues[13] found that patients age less than 30 years old and patients with no prior exposure to lenalidomide therapy have less collection failure. Many studies have found significant demographic parameters in healthy allogeneic donors that affect the success of HSPC mobilization. These include large donor size (eg, weight and body mass index), male sex, race, and preapheresis platelet count.[67]

Underlying patient morbidities may also effect mobilization. Fadini and colleagues[72] found that patients with diabetes have reduced autologous HSPC mobilization using G-CSF with chemotherapy when compared with G-CSF plus plerixafor. It has been hypothesized that diabetes-induced endotheliopathy may have caused compromised integrity of the medullary vascular niche that is critical for HSPC retention and extravasation.

Increased Collection Efficiency with On-Demand or Preemptive Plerixafor

On-demand plerixafor to supplement G-CSF can improve the rate of successful mobilization. As an example, Jantunen and Varmavuo[73] reviewed various published studies and found that the preemptive use of plerixafor on day 5 of G-CSF mobilization when PB CD34 is less than 10/μL improved mobilization. However, determination of the optimal timing and dosing of preemptive plerixafor may further increase the success rate. Storch and colleagues[11] have refined the precollection strategy by determining the PB CD34+ cell concentration on day 4 rather than day 5 of G-CSF mobilization. This early information about PB CD34 provides the capability for real-time clinical decision making regarding the use of plerixafor. Indeed, the use of early plerixafor was associated with a significant decrease in leukapheresis length, blood volume processed, final blood product volume, and non-HSPC cellular impurity (eg, red blood cells and granulocytes). This approach was also confirmed to be logically and operationally advantageous in autologous donors (eg, lymphoma and MM) with low circulating preharvest PB CD34 concentration.[74]

Although the routine use of plerixafor plus G-CSF mobilization may lead to a higher success in mobilization and collection, this combination treatment can be very costly. However, several plerixafor cost analysis studies have been published and suggest that "on-demand" use of plerixafor can actually be cost effective.[75,76] In a high-risk donor or known poor mobilizer, preemptive use of plerixafor can be cost effective by reducing the frequency of remobilization and/or leukapheresis.[14,77]

Optimized Leukapheresis Procedures

The final modifiable parameters to improve stem cell collection efficiency are the volume of blood processed and the type of apheresis equipment used.

Large volume leukapheresis

With the availability of technology that allows for continuous centrifugation and filtration, harvesting the HSPC fraction from a single large volume leukapheresis (LVL) becomes possible. If HSPCs are optimally mobilized, it is feasible to achieve the collection goal within 1 to 2 procedures. However, to accommodate poor mobilizers without excessive numbers of procedures, LVL, which is defined as more than 3 total blood volumes (TBV), has been explored. Several studies have shown that up to 6 TBV can be considered.[78–80] Furthermore, Bojanic and colleagues[78] showed that the quality of the graft, assessed by immunophenotypic markers, remains similar between cells collected over 1 to 4 TBV and 5 to 6 TBV. However, the efficiency of LVL can be variable depending on the donor, apheresis equipment, and apheresis nurse. Additional drawbacks, such as the length of the procedure (up to 5 hours for processing 6 TBV) and the challenge in maintaining a high blood flow rate (ie, catheter clotting). Also, a patient's tolerance to the procedure is another significant clinical concern, because prolonged exposure to citrate anticoagulant may cause hypocalcemia and other electrolyte imbalances.[81] The use of LVL should be determined based on the collection goal, the status of the donor mobilization by PB CD34 count, and the patient's status.

Peripheral blood collection platforms

COBE Spectra (Terumo BCT, Lakewood, CO) has been the most frequently used platform for leukapheresis in the past 2 decades. However, other newer apheresis machines have been developed with improved features to replace the Spectra, such as the Amicus (Fenwal Inc, Lake Zurich, IL) and the Spectra Optia (Terumo BCT). A few studies have been conducted to evaluate these newer models compared with the COBE spectra in both autologous and healthy allogeneic donors. Overall, the successor of the Spectra, the Spectra Optia system, seems to generate a comparable HSPC product with the least amount of red cell contamination, which is clinically beneficial, especially for a major ABO incompatible transplantation. On the other hand, the Amicus platform removes the fewest platelets from the donor, which is a significant consideration in autologous patients with precollection thrombocytopenia. The CD34 yields from these platforms seem to correlate well with the PB CD34 count but the relative performance varies between studies.[82–84] A larger comparative analysis that addresses specific donor cohorts would be helpful to guide the selection of the best apheresis equipment to optimize the HSPC collection process.

LOGISTICAL CONSIDERATIONS DURING STEM CELL COLLECTION

The stem cell collection is logistically complex owing to the number of different services involved (clinical blood and marrow transplant service, apheresis service, flow cytometry laboratory, and stem cell laboratory). Clear communication is required to keep all services aware of donor and product status during the mobilization/collection period, and to ensure the safest and most efficient process.

Prerequisites to Receiving Leukapheresis

Venous line placement
The first step for a successful apheresis procedure is to properly select venous access for the procedure. Considerations should include peripheral versus central access, 2 versus 3 lumens, tunneled versus nontunneled access, and length of time access is needed. Most autologous donors have a central line placed for the duration of the collection. For allogeneic donors, peripheral access may be used if their veins are assessed by an experienced apheresis nurse beforehand.

Preprocedural hematocrit and platelet counts
Autologous donors may have low WBC count, platelet count, and hemoglobin owing to chemotherapy before stem cell collection. Because a large extracorporeal blood volume is required for the leukapheresis procedure, a hematocrit of at least 27% to 28% is desirable before the procedure.[80] Occasionally, a patient may require red blood cell transfusion to reach this goal. Additionally, 35% to 45% of the patient's endogenous platelets can be removed during the apheresis procedure and the magnitude of platelet loss could be contributed to the blood volume processed, specific leukapheresis platform use, and host-specific factors.[85] Therefore, autologous donors should aim to have a minimum of a 20 to 50 $\times$ 10^9/L preprocedural platelet count to prevent possible bleeding complications owing to postprocedural thrombocytopenia.[80]

Adverse Events and Complications of Apheresis

Complications of apheresis for stem cell collection tend to be similar to general complications for therapeutic apheresis, except that the underlying disease in autologous donors may influence the safety and tolerance of the procedure. Donmez and colleagues[86] retrospectively reviewed stem cell collection after 528 mobilization cycles and found an adverse event rate of 13.1% for 1572 procedures. The most common adverse event was numbness of the lips, tongue, or extremities, related to the infused acid citrate dextrose A during the procedure. Multivariate analysis found high amounts of citrate, a greater numbers of procedures, and female gender were associated with the events. Investigators have proposed the administration of prophylactic calcium and intraprocedure ionized calcium monitoring as a solution to this problem.[87] Decreasing the inlet flow rate can also decrease hypocalcemia reactions, but this will also lengthen the procedure time. In addition, heparin may be used for autologous donors receiving LVL who are intolerant to prolonged citrate infusion. Vasovagal/syncope reactions are also relatively common. Allergic reactions, such as burning eyes, periorbital edema, hives, urticarial, wheezing, shortness of breath, hypotension, and tachycardia, can also occur during apheresis procedures. Treatment with diphenhydramine is usually sufficient for minor allergic reactions. Stem cell donors also may report adverse events related to mobilization regimens, such as bone pain related to G-CSF administration or gastrointestinal distress related to plerixafor.

SUMMARY

HSPC mobilization and collection are highly dynamic processes that require interdisciplinary efforts between the clinical service and the apheresis/cell processing services. The use of the PB CD34 count as a predictor for optimal mobilization has greatly improved HSPC collection success; however, the optimal collection strategy still needs to be developed locally based on clinical resources and patient cohorts.

REFERENCES

1. Holig K. G-CSF in healthy allogeneic stem cell donors. Transfus Med Hemother 2013;40(4):225–35.
2. Ozkan MC, Sahin F, Saydam G. Peripheral blood stem cell mobilization from healthy donors. Transfus Apher Sci 2015;53:13–6.
3. Morrison SJ, Scadden DT. The bone marrow niche for haematopoietic stem cells. Nature 2014;505(7483):327–34.
4. Ratajczak MZ, Adamiak M. Membrane lipid rafts, master regulators of hematopoietic stem cell retention in bone marrow and their trafficking. Leukemia 2015;29(7): 1452–7.
5. Wang W, Yu S, Zimmerman G, et al. Notch receptor-ligand engagement maintains hematopoietic stem cell quiescence and niche retention. Stem Cells 2015;33(7):2280–93.
6. Hoggatt J, Pelus LM. Mobilization of hematopoietic stem cells from the bone marrow niche to the blood compartment. Stem Cell Res Ther 2011;2(2):13.
7. Sheppard D, Bredeson C, Allan D, et al. Systematic review of randomized controlled trials of hematopoietic stem cell mobilization strategies for autologous transplantation for hematologic malignancies. Biol Blood Marrow Transplant 2012;18(8):1191–203.
8. Jantunen E, Varmavuo V, Juutilainen A, et al. Kinetics of blood CD34(+) cells after chemotherapy plus G-CSF in poor mobilizers: implications for pre-emptive plerixafor use. Ann Hematol 2012;91(7):1073–9.
9. Douglas KW, Parker AN, Hayden PJ, et al. Plerixafor for PBSC mobilisation in myeloma patients with advanced renal failure: safety and efficacy data in a series of 21 patients from Europe and the USA. Bone Marrow Transplant 2012;47(1): 18–23.
10. Lefrere F, Mauge L, Rea D, et al. A specific time course for mobilization of peripheral blood CD34+ cells after plerixafor injection in very poor mobilizer patients: impact on the timing of the apheresis procedure. Transfusion 2013;53(3):564–9.
11. Storch E, Mark T, Avecilla S, et al. A novel hematopoietic progenitor cell mobilization and collection algorithm based on preemptive CD34 enumeration. Transfusion 2015;55(8):2010–6.
12. Gutensohn K, Magens MM, Kuehnl P, et al. Increasing the economic efficacy of peripheral blood progenitor cell collections by monitoring peripheral blood CD34+ concentrations. Transfusion 2010;50(3):656–62.
13. Duong HK, Bolwell BJ, Rybicki L, et al. Predicting hematopoietic stem cell mobilization failure in patients with multiple myeloma: a simple method using day 1 CD34+ cell yield. J Clin Apher 2011;26(3):111–5.
14. Horwitz ME, Chute JP, Gasparetto C, et al. Preemptive dosing of plerixafor given to poor stem cell mobilizers on day 5 of G-CSF administration. Bone Marrow Transplant 2012;47(8):1051–5.

15. Kotasek D, Shepherd KM, Sage RE, et al. Factors affecting blood stem cell collections following high-dose cyclophosphamide mobilization in lymphoma, myeloma and solid tumors. Bone Marrow Transplant 1992;9(1):11-7.

16. Attal M, Harousseau JL, Stoppa AM, et al. A prospective, randomized trial of autologous bone marrow transplantation and chemotherapy in multiple myeloma. Intergroupe Francais du Myelome. N Engl J Med 1996;335(2):91-7.

17. Jantunen E, Putkonen M, Nousiainen T, et al. Low-dose or intermediate-dose cyclophosphamide plus granulocyte colony-stimulating factor for progenitor cell mobilisation in patients with multiple myeloma. Bone Marrow Transplant 2003;31(5):347-51.

18. Mueller BU, Keller S, Seipel K, et al. Stem cell mobilization chemotherapy with gemcitabine is effective and safe in myeloma patients with bortezomib induced neurotoxicity. Leuk Lymphoma 2015;1-28.

19. Antar A, Otrock ZK, Kharfan-Dabaja MA, et al. G-CSF plus preemptive plerixafor vs hyperfractionated CY plus G-CSF for autologous stem cell mobilization in multiple myeloma: effectiveness, safety and cost analysis. Bone Marrow Transplant 2015;50(6):813-7.

20. Giralt S, Costa L, Schriber J, et al. Optimizing autologous stem cell mobilization strategies to improve patient outcomes: consensus guidelines and recommendations. Biol Blood Marrow Transplant 2014;20(3):295-308.

21. Damon LE, Damon LE. Mobilization of hematopoietic stem cells into the peripheral blood. Expert Rev Hematol 2009;2(6):717-33.

22. Martino M, Laszlo D, Lanza F. Long-active granulocyte colony-stimulating factor for peripheral blood hematopoietic progenitor cell mobilization. Expert Opin Biol Ther 2014;14(6):757-72.

23. Kim MG, Han N, Lee EK, et al. Pegfilgrastim vs filgrastim in PBSC mobilization for autologous hematopoietic SCT: a systematic review and meta-analysis. Bone Marrow Transplant 2015;50(4):523-30.

24. Ataergin S, Arpaci F, Turan M, et al. Reduced dose of lenograstim is as efficacious as standard dose of filgrastim for peripheral blood stem cell mobilization and transplantation: a randomized study in patients undergoing autologous peripheral stem cell transplantation. Am J Hematol 2008;83(8):644-8.

25. Kuderer NM, Dale DC, Crawford J, et al. Impact of primary prophylaxis with granulocyte colony-stimulating factor on febrile neutropenia and mortality in adult cancer patients receiving chemotherapy: a systematic review. J Clin Oncol 2007;25(21):3158-67.

26. Kopf B, De Giorgi U, Vertogen B, et al. A randomized study comparing filgrastim versus lenograstim versus molgramostim plus chemotherapy for peripheral blood progenitor cell mobilization. Bone Marrow Transplant 2006;38(6):407-12.

27. Kuan JW, Su AT, Wong SP, et al. A randomized double blind control trial comparing filgrastim and pegfilgrastim in cyclophosphamide peripheral blood hematopoietic stem cell mobilization. Transfus Apher Sci 2015;53:196-204.

28. Ria R, Reale A, Melaccio A, et al. Filgrastim, lenograstim and pegfilgrastim in the mobilization of peripheral blood progenitor cells in patients with lymphoproliferative malignancies. Clin Exp Med 2015;15(2):145-50.

29. Pham T, Patil S, Fleming S, et al. Comparison of biosimilar filgrastim with originator filgrastim for peripheral blood stem cell mobilization and engraftment in patients with multiple myeloma undergoing autologous stem cell transplantation. Transfusion 2015;55:2709-13.

30. Schmitt M, Xu X, Hilgendorf I, et al. Mobilization of PBSC for allogeneic transplantation by the use of the G-CSF biosimilar XM02 in healthy donors. Bone Marrow Transplant 2013;48(7):922–5.
31. Manko J, Walter-Croneck A, Jawniak D, et al. A clinical comparison of the efficacy and safety of biosimilar G-CSF and originator G-CSF in haematopoietic stem cell mobilization. Pharmacol Rep 2014;66(2):239–42.
32. Lane TA, Law P, Maruyama M, et al. Harvesting and enrichment of hematopoietic progenitor cells mobilized into the peripheral blood of normal donors by granulocyte-macrophage colony-stimulating factor (GM-CSF) or G-CSF: potential role in allogeneic marrow transplantation. Blood 1995;85(1):275–82.
33. Weaver CH, Schulman KA, Wilson-Relyea B, et al. Randomized trial of filgrastim, sargramostim, or sequential sargramostim and filgrastim after myelosuppressive chemotherapy for the harvesting of peripheral-blood stem cells. J Clin Oncol 2000;18(1):43–53.
34. Arora M, Burns LJ, Barker JN, et al. Randomized comparison of granulocyte colony-stimulating factor versus granulocyte-macrophage colony-stimulating factor plus intensive chemotherapy for peripheral blood stem cell mobilization and autologous transplantation in multiple myeloma. Biol Blood Marrow Transplant 2004;10(6):395–404.
35. Bregni M, Siena S, Di Nicola M, et al. Comparative effects of granulocyte-macrophage colony-stimulating factor and granulocyte colony-stimulating factor after high-dose cyclophosphamide cancer therapy. J Clin Oncol 1996;14(2):628–35.
36. Quittet P, Ceballos P, Lopez E, et al. Low doses of GM-CSF (molgramostim) and G-CSF (filgrastim) after cyclophosphamide (4 g/m2) enhance the peripheral blood progenitor cell harvest: results of two randomized studies including 120 patients. Bone Marrow Transplant 2006;38(4):275–84.
37. De Clercq E. The AMD3100 story: the path to the discovery of a stem cell mobilizer (Mozobil). Biochem Pharmacol 2009;77(11):1655–64.
38. De Clercq E, Yamamoto N, Pauwels R, et al. Potent and selective inhibition of human immunodeficiency virus (HIV)-1 and HIV-2 replication by a class of bicyclams interacting with a viral uncoating event. Proc Natl Acad Sci U S A 1992;89(12):5286–90.
39. DiPersio JF, Micallef IN, Stiff PJ, et al. Phase III prospective randomized double-blind placebo-controlled trial of plerixafor plus granulocyte colony-stimulating factor compared with placebo plus granulocyte colony-stimulating factor for autologous stem-cell mobilization and transplantation for patients with non-Hodgkin's lymphoma. J Clin Oncol 2009;27(28):4767–73.
40. DiPersio JF, Stadtmauer EA, Nademanee A, et al. Plerixafor and G-CSF versus placebo and G-CSF to mobilize hematopoietic stem cells for autologous stem cell transplantation in patients with multiple myeloma. Blood 2009;113(23):5720–6.
41. Kumar SK, Mikhael J, Laplant B, et al. Phase 2 trial of intravenously administered plerixafor for stem cell mobilization in patients with multiple myeloma following lenalidomide-based initial therapy. Bone Marrow Transplant 2014;49(2):201–5.
42. Hubel K, Fresen MM, Salwender H, et al. Plerixafor with and without chemotherapy in poor mobilizers: results from the German compassionate use program. Bone Marrow Transplant 2011;46(8):1045–52.
43. Devine SM, Vij R, Rettig M, et al. Rapid mobilization of functional donor hematopoietic cells without G-CSF using AMD3100, an antagonist of the CXCR4/SDF-1 interaction. Blood 2008;112(4):990–8.

44. Girbl T, Lunzer V, Greil R, et al. The CXCR4 and adhesion molecule expression of CD34+ hematopoietic cells mobilized by "on-demand" addition of plerixafor to granulocyte-colony-stimulating factor. Transfusion 2014;54(9):2325–35.

45. Valtola J, Varmavuo V, Ropponen A, et al. Blood graft cellular composition and posttransplant recovery in non-Hodgkin's lymphoma patients mobilized with or without plerixafor: a prospective comparison. Transfusion 2015;55:2358–68.

46. Ding L, Saunders TL, Enikolopov G, et al. Endothelial and perivascular cells maintain haematopoietic stem cells. Nature 2012;481(7382):457–62.

47. Shpall EJ, Wheeler CA, Turner SA, et al. A randomized phase 3 study of peripheral blood progenitor cell mobilization with stem cell factor and filgrastim in high-risk breast cancer patients. Blood 1999;93(8):2491–501.

48. Lapierre V, Rossi JF, Heshmati F, et al. Ancestim (r-metHuSCF) plus filgrastim and/or chemotherapy for mobilization of blood progenitors in 513 poorly mobilizing cancer patients: the French compassionate experience. Bone Marrow Transplant 2011;46(7):936–42.

49. Johnsen HE, Geisler C, Juvonen E, et al. Priming with r-metHuSCF and filgrastim or chemotherapy and filgrastim in patients with malignant lymphomas: a randomized phase II pilot study of mobilization and engraftment. Bone Marrow Transplant 2011;46(1):44–51.

50. Papayannopoulou T, Nakamoto B. Peripheralization of hemopoietic progenitors in primates treated with anti-VLA4 integrin. Proc Natl Acad Sci U S A 1993;90(20):9374–8.

51. Meehan KR, Areman EM, Ericson SG, et al. Mobilization, collection, and processing of autologous peripheral blood stem cells: development of a clinical process with associated costs. J Hematother Stem Cell Res 2000;9(5):767–71.

52. Weaver CH, Hazelton B, Birch R, et al. An analysis of engraftment kinetics as a function of the CD34 content of peripheral blood progenitor cell collections in 692 patients after the administration of myeloablative chemotherapy. Blood 1995;86(10):3961–9.

53. Carral A, de la Rubia J, Martin G, et al. Factors influencing hematopoietic recovery after autologous blood stem cell transplantation in patients with acute myeloblastic leukemia and with non-myeloid malignancies. Bone Marrow Transplant 2002;29(10):825–32.

54. Schots R, Van Riet I, Damiaens S, et al. The absolute number of circulating CD34+ cells predicts the number of hematopoietic stem cells that can be collected by apheresis. Bone Marrow Transplant 1996;17(4):509–15.

55. Yu J, Leisenring W, Bensinger WI, et al. The predictive value of white cell or CD34+ cell count in the peripheral blood for timing apheresis and maximizing yield. Transfusion 1999;39(5):442–50.

56. Gambell P, Herbert K, Dickinson M, et al. Peripheral blood CD34+ cell enumeration as a predictor of apheresis yield: an analysis of more than 1,000 collections. Biol Blood Marrow Transplant 2012;18(5):763–72.

57. Lefrere F, Zohar S, Beaudier S, et al. Evaluation of an algorithm based on peripheral blood hematopoietic progenitor cell and CD34+ cell concentrations to optimize peripheral blood progenitor cell collection by apheresis. Transfusion 2007;47(10):1851–7.

58. Padmanabhan A, Reich-Slotky R, Jhang JS, et al. Use of the haematopoietic progenitor cell parameter in optimizing timing of peripheral blood stem cell harvest. Vox Sang 2009;97(2):153–9.

59. Letestu R, Marzac C, Audat F, et al. Use of hematopoietic progenitor cell count on the Sysmex XE-2100 for peripheral blood stem cell harvest monitoring. Leuk Lymphoma 2007;48(1):89–96.

60. Villa CH, Shore T, Van Besien K, et al. Addition of plerixafor to mobilization regimens in autologous peripheral blood stem cell transplants does not affect the correlation of preharvest hematopoietic precursor cell enumeration with first-harvest CD34+ stem cell yield. Biol Blood Marrow Transplant 2012;18(12):1867–75.

61. Ford CD, Pace N, Lehman C. Factors affecting the efficiency of collection of CD34-positive peripheral blood cells by a blood cell separator. Transfusion 1998;38(11–12):1046–50.

62. Verlinden A, Van de Velde A, Verpooten GA, et al. Determining factors predictive of CD34+ cell collection efficiency in an effort to avoid extended and repeated apheresis sessions. J Clin Apher 2013;28(6):404–10.

63. Elliott C, Samson DM, Armitage S, et al. When to harvest peripheral-blood stem cells after mobilization therapy: prediction of CD34-positive cell yield by preceding day CD34-positive concentration in peripheral blood. J Clin Oncol 1996;14(3):970–3.

64. Ho AD, Gluck S, Germond C, et al. Optimal timing for collections of blood progenitor cells following induction chemotherapy and granulocyte-macrophage colony-stimulating factor for autologous transplantation in advanced breast cancer. Leukemia 1993;7(11):1738–46.

65. Makar RS, Padmanabhan A, Kim HC, et al. Use of laboratory tests to guide initiation of autologous hematopoietic progenitor cell collection by apheresis: results from the multicenter hematopoietic progenitor cell collection by Apheresis Laboratory Trigger Survey. Transfus Med Rev 2014;28(4):198–204.

66. Sutherland DR. Assessment of peripheral blood stem cell grafts by CD34+ cell enumeration: toward a standardized flow cytometric approach. J Hematother 1996;5(3):209–10.

67. Teipel R, Schetelig J, Kramer M, et al. Prediction of hematopoietic stem cell yield after mobilization with granulocyte-colony-stimulating factor in healthy unrelated donors. Transfusion 2015;55:2855–63.

68. Anguita-Compagnon AT, Dibarrart MT, Palma J, et al. Mobilization and collection of peripheral blood stem cells: guidelines for blood volume to process, based on CD34-positive blood cell count in adults and children. Transplant Proc 2010;42(1):339–44.

69. Schade H, Chhabra S, Kang Y, et al. Similar dynamics of intraapheresis autologous CD34+ recruitment and collection efficiency in patients undergoing mobilization with or without plerixafor. Transfusion 2014;54(12):3131–7.

70. Tanosaki R, Kumazawa T, Yoshida A, et al. Novel and rapid enumeration method of peripheral blood stem cells using automated hematology analyzer. Int J Lab Hematol 2014;36(5):521–30.

71. Jantunen E, Kuittinen T, Nousiainen T. Is chemotherapy scoring useful to predict progenitor cell mobilisation in patients with non-Hodgkin's lymphoma? Bone Marrow Transplant 2003;32(6):569–73.

72. Fadini GP, Fiala M, Cappellari R, et al. Diabetes limits stem cell mobilization following G-CSF but not Plerixafor. Diabetes 2015;64(8):2969–77.

73. Jantunen E, Varmavuo V. Plerixafor for mobilization of blood stem cells in autologous transplantation: an update. Expert Opin Biol Ther 2014;14(6):851–61.

74. Sanchez-Ortega I, Querol S, Encuentra M, et al. Plerixafor in patients with lymphoma and multiple myeloma: effectiveness in cases with very low circulating

CD34+ cell levels and preemptive intervention vs remobilization. Bone Marrow Transplant 2015;50(1):34–9.

75. Milone G, Martino M, Spadaro A, et al. Plerixafor on-demand combined with chemotherapy and granulocyte colony-stimulating factor: significant improvement in peripheral blood stem cells mobilization and harvest with no increase in costs. Br J Haematol 2014;164(1):113–23.

76. Micallef IN, Sinha S, Gastineau DA, et al. Cost-effectiveness analysis of a risk-adapted algorithm of plerixafor use for autologous peripheral blood stem cell mobilization. Biol Blood Marrow Transplant 2013;19(1):87–93.

77. Li J, Hamilton E, Vaughn L, et al. Effectiveness and cost analysis of "just-in-time" salvage plerixafor administration in autologous transplant patients with poor stem cell mobilization kinetics. Transfusion 2011;51(10):2175–82.

78. Bojanic I, Dubravcic K, Batinic D, et al. Large volume leukapheresis: efficacy and safety of processing patient's total blood volume six times. Transfus Apher Sci 2011;44(2):139–47.

79. Majado MJ, Minguela A, Gonzalez-Garcia C, et al. Large-volume-apheresis facilitates autologous transplantation of hematopoietic progenitors in poor mobilizer patients. J Clin Apher 2009;24(1):12–7.

80. Gasova Z, Bhuiyan-Ludvikova Z, Bohmova M, et al. PBPC collections: management, techniques and risks. Transfus Apher Sci 2010;43(2):237–43.

81. Humpe A, Riggert J, Munzel U, et al. A prospective, randomized, sequential crossover trial of large-volume versus normal-volume leukapheresis procedures: effects on serum electrolytes, platelet counts, and other coagulation measures. Transfusion 2000;40(3):368–74.

82. Steininger PA, Strasser EF, Weiss D, et al. First comparative evaluation of a new leukapheresis technology in non-cytokine-stimulated donors. Vox Sang 2014; 106(3):248–55.

83. Brauninger S, Bialleck H, Thorausch K, et al. Allogeneic donor peripheral blood "stem cell" apheresis: prospective comparison of two apheresis systems. Transfusion 2012;52(5):1137–45.

84. Wu FY, Heng KK, Salleh RB, et al. Comparing peripheral blood stem cell collection using the COBE Spectra, Haemonetics MCS+, and Baxter Amicus. Transfus Apher Sci 2012;47(3):345–50.

85. Miller JP, Perry EH, Price TH, et al. Recovery and safety profiles of marrow and PBSC donors: experience of the National Marrow Donor Program. Biol Blood Marrow Transplant 2008;14(9 Suppl):29–36.

86. Donmez A, Arik B, Tombuloglu M, et al. Risk factors for adverse events during collection of peripheral blood stem cells. Transfus Apher Sci 2011;45(1):13–6.

87. Buchta C, Macher M, Bieglmayer C, et al. Reduction of adverse citrate reactions during autologous large-volume PBPC apheresis by continuous infusion of calcium-gluconate. Transfusion 2003;43(11):1615–21.

Management of Patients with Sickle Cell Disease Using Transfusion Therapy
Guidelines and Complications

Stella T. Chou, MD[a],*, Ross M. Fasano, MD[b],*

KEYWORDS

- Sickle cell disease • Red blood cell transfusion • Alloimmunization • Iron overload

KEY POINTS

- Urgent or emergent red blood cell transfusion is indicated for acute ischemic stroke, acute chest syndrome, splenic or hepatic sequestration, transient aplastic crisis, multisystem organ failure, intrahepatic cholestasis, or obstetric complications in patients with sickle cell disease (SCD).
- Chronic transfusion therapy is indicated for primary and secondary stroke prevention and short-term for prevention of splenic sequestration recurrence.
- Patients with SCD should receive red cells antigen matched for C, E, and K to reduce alloimmunization risk.
- The iron status of chronically transfused patients with SCD should be closely monitored and iron chelation therapy and/or erythrocytapheresis implemented to maintain iron balance.

INTRODUCTION

Over the past few decades, significant advances in the care of patients with sickle cell disease (SCD) have led to improvements in morbidity and survival. The average life span of patients with SCD has increased from 14 years in 1973 to more than 50 years.[1] A key component in the management of patients with SCD is red blood cell (RBC)

[a] Department of Pediatrics, Abramson Research Center, The Children's Hospital of Philadelphia, Perelman School of Medicine, University of Pennsylvania, 316D, 3615 Civic Center Boulevard, Philadelphia, PA 19104, USA; [b] Transfusion, Tissue, & Apheresis, Children's Healthcare of Atlanta and Grady Health System Transfusion Services, Departments of Clinical Pathology and Pediatric Hematology, Emory University School of Medicine, 7105B Woodruff Memorial Building, 101 Woodruff Circle, Atlanta, GA 30322, USA
* Corresponding author. Department of Clinical Pathology, Emory University School of Medicine, 7105B Woodruff Memorial Building, 101 Woodruff Circle, Atlanta, GA 30322
E-mail addresses: chous@email.chop.edu; ross.fasano@emory.edu

Hematol Oncol Clin N Am 30 (2016) 591–608
http://dx.doi.org/10.1016/j.hoc.2016.01.011
0889-8588/16/$ – see front matter © 2016 Elsevier Inc. All rights reserved.

transfusion therapy. The major goals of RBC transfusions are relief of anemia, reduction of circulating sickle hemoglobin (HbS) erythrocytes, and improvement in oxygen-carrying capacity.[2] Although transfusion can be lifesaving, it is not without adverse effects. Using evidence-based transfusion policies can minimize transfusion-related complications. This review addresses RBC transfusion methods, indications (**Table 1**), and complications.

METHODS OF TRANSFUSION THERAPY

RBC transfusions can be administered by simple or exchange transfusion. Exchange transfusion is preferably performed by automated erythrocytapheresis but can be performed manually. Simple transfusions are dosed in units (1–3 units for adults) or

Table 1
Indications for transfusion therapy in adults and children with sickle cell disease

Transfusion Indication	Transfusion Method
Generally accepted indications for transfusion	
Acute ischemic stroke	Exchange transfusion preferred
Primary stroke prevention	Chronic simple or exchange transfusion[a]
Secondary stroke prevention	Chronic simple or exchange transfusion[a]
Acute chest syndrome (acute)	Simple or exchange transfusion[a]
Acute splenic sequestration	Simple transfusion
Acute splenic sequestration, recurrence	Chronic simple transfusion (before splenectomy)[b]
Preoperative (when general anesthesia required)	Simple transfusion
Transient aplastic crisis	Simple transfusion
Acute multisystem organ failure	Simple or exchange transfusion[c]
Acute hepatic sequestration	Simple or exchange transfusion[c]
Acute intrahepatic cholestasis	Simple or exchange transfusion[c]
Acute sickle or obstetric complications during pregnancy	Simple or exchange transfusion[c]
Controversial indications for transfusion	
Acute chest syndrome (recurrent)	Chronic simple or exchange transfusion[c]
Vasoocclusive painful episode (recurrent)	Chronic simple or exchange transfusion[c]
Pulmonary hypertension	Chronic simple or exchange transfusion[c]
Transfusion generally not indicated	
Uncomplicated vasoocclusive painful episode	NA
Priapism	NA
Uncomplicated pregnancy	NA
Leg ulcers	NA
Nonsurgically managed avascular necrosis	NA

Abbreviation: NA, not applicable.
   [a] Exchange transfusion may be preferred in rapidly deteriorating patients when emergent HbS reduction is needed or when there are concerns for post-transfusion hyperviscosity due to a high pretransfusion hemoglobin (ie, >9 g/dL).
   [b] Chronic transfusion may be used to delay but not prevent the need for splenectomy in very young children (ie, <2 years) who are at increased risk for invasive pneumococcal infections.
   [c] Exchange transfusion may be preferred in patients with iron overload.

volume (10–20 mL/kg for children). Exchange transfusion requires a higher volume of RBCs administered (1.0–1.5 × patients' RBC volume) but simultaneously removes patients' RBCs. Erythrocytapheresis offers the advantage of rapidly reducing HbS independent of the hematocrit and minimizes iron accumulation. Exchange transfusion is often preferred for emergent HbS reduction in patients with higher pretransfusion hemoglobin (Hb)(>9 g/dL) because of hyperviscosity concerns and to prevent iron overload. The decision to use simple versus exchange transfusion depends on specific clinical needs and availability of resources, including apheresis equipment and technical support, adequate supply of antigen-negative donor units, and the potential need for central venous access.[3–5] Partial manual exchange (PME) is an alternative method for patients with a higher Hb (>8.5 g/dL) and involves phlebotomy of 5 to 10 mL/kg (depending on patients' baseline Hb and tolerance) immediately before transfusion. PME has been used to slow progression of transfusional iron overload when used as a chronic transfusion regimen.[6]

INDICATIONS
Acute Splenic Sequestration

RBC transfusion is indicated for acute exacerbation of anemia occurring with splenic sequestration. Because splenic involution is usually complete by 5 years of age in hemoglobin SS and Sβ° thalassemia, acute splenic sequestration most commonly affects young children. The spleen becomes acutely engorged with sequestered blood and may result in a precipitous decrease in Hb level. Severe episodes may lead to hypovolemic shock and death from cardiovascular collapse within hours. Immediate RBC transfusion will correct the anemia and hypovolemia, but patients should be transfused cautiously to prevent hyperviscosity after splenic sequestration resolves. Aliquots of 5 mL/kg may be administered along with close monitoring of the spleen size, Hb level, and cardiovascular status. In cases of severe sequestration and anemia with hypovolemic shock, initial transfusion with 10 mL/kg packed RBCs (PRBCs) is appropriate. Relapse of acute splenic sequestration is frequent, with 50% to 75% of patients experiencing recurrent episodes.[7] Chronic RBC transfusion to prevent recurrence has not been prospectively studied but is often used to delay definitive treatment of splenectomy in very young children. In a retrospective multicenter study of 190 children with hemoglobin-SS or Sβ° disease, 29% were managed with a blood transfusion program and, overall, 37% ultimately required splenectomy.[7] However, 54% of patients were managed with close monitoring and without prophylactic blood transfusion or splenectomy, of which 59% did not experience a recurrent episode.

Transient Aplastic Crisis

Human parvovirus B19 infects erythrocyte precursors and temporarily suppresses erythropoiesis that can result in severe anemia given the shortened life span of RBCs in patients with SCD. In a single-institution observational study of parvovirus B19–induced red cell aplasia, the median nadir Hb was 4.8 g/dL and 49 of 68 pediatric patients (72%) received a transfusion.[8] The need for transfusion depends on the severity of the anemia, whether they are in the reticulocytopenia stage, and the clinical status of patients. Because anemia associated with red cell aplasia is subacute, patients are typically euvolemic and physiologically compensated. RBC transfusion should be administered slowly with serial small aliquots to prevent congestive heart failure. Parvovirus aplastic crisis typically does not recur because of long-term humoral immunity.

Acute Chest Syndrome

Acute chest syndrome (ACS) describes a new pulmonary infiltrate and respiratory findings, including cough, dyspnea, or new-onset hypoxia, in patients with SCD and is often accompanied by fever. Triggers include infection, pulmonary fat embolism, hypoventilation/atelectasis, and bronchospasm. ACS is the leading cause of death and second most common cause of hospitalization among patients with SCD. The management is primarily supportive and includes respiratory therapy, antibiotics, and, often, RBC transfusion. There have been no randomized controlled trials comparing either simple or exchange transfusion versus no transfusion for ACS. However, in a large epidemiologic study of ACS, transfusion was associated with a shorter duration of hospitalization, suggesting an association with clinical improvement.[9] A difference in efficacy of simple transfusion compared with exchange transfusion as measured by length of hospital stay was not detected in a small study of 20 patients with ACS.[10] In practice, simple transfusion should be considered for any patient with ACS and hypoxemia or acute exacerbation of anemia. Exchange transfusion is typically reserved for patients who are not sufficiently anemic to accommodate a simple transfusion or those with progressive respiratory decline or persistent hypoxia despite oxygen supplementation or simple transfusion.

No prospective randomized trial has been performed to determine the efficacy of chronic transfusion therapy to prevent recurrent ACS. Chronic transfusion therapy is sometimes offered, particularly to individuals who experienced a severe or life-threatening episode. A dramatic reduction in hospitalization for ACS was observed in children undergoing chronic transfusion for primary stroke prevention compared with the observed group, suggesting chronic transfusions may prevent recurrent episodes.[11] In one single-institution study, chronic transfusion therapy reduced the incidence of ACS events among patients with recurrent ACS but did not significantly impact episode severity.[12] Although hydroxyurea is indicated for the prevention of recurrent ACS,[13] future studies are needed to compare chronic transfusion therapy and hydroxyurea for recurrent ACS prevention.

Acute Sickle Hepatopathy

Acute hepatic sequestration and sickle cell intrahepatic cholestasis (SCIC) are severe forms of hepatic injury from vascular occlusion of liver sinusoids.[14] Acute hepatic sequestration manifests as painful enlarging hepatomegaly with a concurrent decrease in hematocrit, reticulocytosis, direct hyperbilirubinemia, and mild transaminitis. Although acute hepatic sequestration rarely results in end organ failure, simple or exchange transfusion is often necessary to resolve the hepatopathy and anemia.[15] However, overly aggressive simple transfusion should be avoided to prevent acute hyperviscosity syndrome resulting from rapid release of intrahepatic RBCs back into the circulation with resolved sequestration.

SCIC is the most severe form of acute sickle hepatopathy, with an overall mortality rate of 40% to 50% in adults and 30% in children due to uncontrolled bleeding and fulminant liver failure.[14] SCIC manifests with sudden onset of right upper quadrant abdominal pain, significantly elevated transaminases (>1000 mg/dL), severe hyperbilirubinemia (total serum bilirubin often >50 mg/dL), coagulopathy, hepatomegaly, renal insufficiency, and acute liver failure in severe cases.[16] Patients can have recurrent episodes, and a subset develop chronic progressive disease that evolves into progressive liver failure.[17] Limited reports describe outcomes based on transfusion management. Ahn and colleagues[18] reviewed 22 cases (7 pediatric, 15 adults) of severe sickle hepatopathy in the literature that met criteria for SCIC; 7 of 9 patients who received exchange transfusion survived compared with 1 of 13 patients who did not receive erythrocytapheresis. Although this data set is limited, it supports a role for exchange transfusion in the management of SCIC, particularly acute SCIC.[15,17] Correction of coagulopathies with plasma, cryoprecipitate, and platelet transfusions is also often necessary. Maintaining HbS levels less than 30% by chronic erythrocytapheresis has been proposed for patients with recurrent episodes of acute SCIC or chronic progressive hepatopathy.[17]

Multisystem Organ Failure

Multisystem organ failure (MSOF) is a life-threatening complication of SCD resulting from diffuse microvascular occlusion, which usually develops several days after a severe vasoocclusive crisis (VOC). MSOF is characterized by rapid lung, liver, and/or kidney dysfunction and is typically accompanied by a precipitous decrease in the Hb level and platelet count, fever, encephalopathy, and rhabdomyolysis. In addition to broad-spectrum antibiotics, mechanical ventilation, pharmacologic and/or mechanical hemodynamic support, and renal replacement therapy, the use of RBC transfusion can be life saving. The largest retrospective report of SCD-associated MSOF included 17 episodes occurring after unusually severe VOCs.[19] All patients except one recovered with aggressive transfusion support via either multiple simple transfusions or an exchange transfusion. The National Heart, Lung, and Blood Institute (NHLBI)–appointed SCD expert panel recommends immediate simple or exchange transfusion for MSOF because of the gravity of this severe sickle-related manifestation.[15]

Preoperative Transfusion Management

Perioperative conditions, including suboptimal hydration, poor oxygenation, and acidemia, can lead to SCD-related complications, such as ACS, painful VOC, and infections. The Transfusion Alternatives Preoperatively in SCD (TAPS) trial demonstrated that preoperative transfusion is associated with decreased perioperative complications.[20] The TAPS trial compared outcomes of preoperative transfusion versus no transfusion in patients with HbSS or undergoing low-risk or medium-risk surgery. The study was terminated early because of an imbalance of adverse events occurring in the no-preoperative-transfusion arm, with 13 of 33 (39%) individuals experiencing a clinically important complication compared with 5 of 34 (15%) patients who were transfused preoperatively. Ten of 11 serious adverse events were ACS: 9 in the no transfusion and one in the transfusion group. The trial did not include individuals with hemoglobin SC or Sβ$^+$ thalassemia, and poor enrollment of patients requiring low-risk procedures hampered the determination of optimal management for this surgical category.[20] A prior randomized control trial showed that preoperative simple transfusion to achieve a Hb of 10 g/dL is equally effective in preventing postoperative complications compared with erythrocytapheresis to decrease the HbS level to less than 30%.[21] Taken together, patients with SCD should receive a simple transfusion preoperatively to increase the Hb to 10 g/dL for medium- to high-risk surgery.

Neurologic Complications

In children with SCD, the routine use of transcranial Doppler (TCD) screening coupled with chronic transfusion therapy has decreased the prevalence of overt stroke from 11% to 1%.[22] However, neurologic complications in children and adults with SCD remain a major cause of long-term morbidity. Acute ischemic stroke is managed with RBC transfusion to reduce the HbS level to less than 30% to prevent progression of cerebral ischemia. Exchange transfusion at the time of stroke presentation may be associated with a lower risk of subsequent stroke compared with simple transfusion,[23] but no prospective study has directly addressed this question. In practice, erythrocytapheresis is the preferred transfusion method for initial treatment of an acute stroke. A simple transfusion may be considered for immediate treatment because it may require several hours to establish central venous access, crossmatch multiple PRBC units, and mobilize the apheresis team for erythrocytapheresis.

An evidence-based approach to the management of acute hemorrhagic stroke in patients with SCD is lacking.[22,24] In the largest case series, 15 adults with SCD with subarachnoid hemorrhage from ruptured intracranial aneurysms were treated with partial exchange transfusion in the acute setting before cerebral angiography.[25] Given the lack of formal studies to guide management of hemorrhagic strokes in individuals with SCD, transfusion in the acute setting to decrease the HbS to less than 30% is recommended in addition to therapy for acute intracranial hemorrhage for the general population, including blood pressure management and seizure control.[22,24]

Stroke recurs in 60% to 90% of patients without therapeutic intervention[26] and decreases to approximately 20% with chronic RBC transfusions when the HbS is maintained at less than 30%.[27,28] Although a controlled clinical trial is lacking, standard care for secondary stroke prevention is chronic transfusion therapy. Indefinite therapy is recommended, as discontinuation after short-term or long-term prophylactic transfusions has led to recurrent stroke, even with transition to hydroxyurea.[29] The randomized phase 3 trial, Stroke With Transfusions Changing to Hydroxyurea, addressed transition to hydroxyurea for patients with a history of stroke and iron overload. The trial was closed because of statistical futility on the composite end point of iron overload resolution and stroke prevention. At the time of study closure, no strokes occurred in patients receiving transfusions with chelation, but 7 patients (10%) receiving hydroxyurea and phlebotomy had a new stroke. Moreover, patients receiving chronic transfusion for secondary stroke prevention are still at risk for silent cerebral infarcts (SCIs),[27,30] and cerebral vasculopathy progression.[27,31,32] Taken together, transfusion remains the optimal choice for managing individuals with SCD and stroke.

Children with SCD at the highest risk of overt stroke can be identified by abnormally high blood flow velocities on TCD ultrasound. The Stroke Prevention Trial for sickle cell anemia study (STOP) demonstrated that chronic transfusion therapy decreased the rate of initial stroke in children with an abnormal TCD by 92% compared with the observation arm.[33] Transfusion reduces cerebral blood-flow velocities, in part because of correction of the anemia, which contributes to lower stroke risk. Universal adoption of routine TCD screening and primary prophylactic transfusion therapy for at-risk patients has resulted in significantly decreased rates of first stroke.[34–36] The STOP2 trial supported the use of chronic transfusion indefinitely, as discontinuation after 30 months resulted in an increased rate of abnormal TCD conversion and overt stroke as well as a higher occurrence of SCIs.[37,38]

Based on previous studies demonstrating that hydroxyurea can lower TCD velocities in patients with SCD,[39,40] the Transfusions Changing to Hydroxyurea (TWiTCH) trial (ClinicalTrials.gov: NCT01425307) aimed to compare the efficacy of hydroxyurea with transfusion therapy for children with abnormal TCDs but no primary stroke. The TWiTCH study ended in 2014 at the first interim analysis after data indicated the trial had reached its primary end point; preliminary results showed that hydroxyurea is not inferior to chronic RBC transfusion in lowering TCD velocities in children with abnormal

TCDs. Given the burden of chronic transfusion therapy and because most children with abnormal TCDs will not have a stroke if untreated, the ability to prevent stroke with hydroxyurea is a significant advance.

SCI is more common than overt stroke and is associated with increased risk of overt stroke, new or enlarged SCIs, poor academic achievement, and lower IQ.[41–43] The Silent Infarct Transfusion trial demonstrated that chronic transfusion therapy significantly reduced the incidence of recurrent cerebral infarcts in patients with SCIs at baseline, no history of overt stroke, and normal TCD velocities.[44] Notably, 6 of 99 children (6%) assigned to transfusions had an event (1 stroke, 5 new or enlarged SCIs) compared with 14 of 97 children (14%) in the observation group (7 strokes, 7 new of enlarged SCIs). Because approximately 25% of children with SCD have SCIs,[42,45] the resources needed to provide chronic transfusions to this group would be immense. Whether hydroxyurea can prevent new SCIs or overt stroke in patients with SCIs is not known. Future studies are also needed to determine whether patients with magnetic resonance angiography–defined vasculopathy but normal TCD velocities would benefit from RBC transfusions to prevent vasculopathy progression and/or silent or overt strokes.

CONTROVERSIAL INDICATIONS
Pulmonary Hypertension

Pulmonary arterial hypertension (PAH) is a common complication in adults with SCD and imposes an increased risk of death. The incidence of PAH diagnosed by right heart catheterization (RHC) is between 6% and 11% in adults with SCD.[46–48] Mortality in these patients is approximately 35% to 40% at 3 to 6 years from diagnosis.[47,48] RHC is the gold standard for diagnosing PAH; but noninvasive evaluations, including tricuspid regurgitant jet velocity (TRV) by Doppler echocardiography, serum N-terminal pro–brain natriuretic peptide (NT-pro-BNP), and the 6-minute walk distance, can be used to predict the presence of PAH and estimate mortality risk.

There are no randomized control trials of hydroxyurea or transfusion therapy for patients with SCD and PAH. The American Thoracic Society (ATS) recommends hydroxyurea for all patients with HbSS who have a TRV of 3.0 m/s or greater alone or TRV of greater than 2.5 m/s with either an elevated NT-pro-BNP level or RHC-confirmed PAH based on studies showing the benefits of hydroxyurea in reducing morbidity and mortality in SCD.[49,50] Transfusion may prevent chronic regional pulmonary hypoxia by reducing the frequency of ACS and decreasing nitric oxide depletion, which results from chronic hemolysis, both of which are risk factors for PAH in SCD.[51] Because transfusion may reverse or stabilize PAH in its early stages by mitigating these pulmonary endothelial effects, the ATS recommends that chronic transfusion therapy be offered to patients who are not responsive to or not candidates for hydroxyurea.[51,52] A recent cross-sectional study of children and young adults with HbSS or HbSβ° supports this recommendation by demonstrating a protective effect of chronic transfusions on pulmonary vascular disease defined by lower TRV measurements.[53] Further investigation is needed to determine if either chronic transfusions or hydroxyurea impact mortality.

Pregnancy in Sickle Cell Disease

Pregnant women with SCD have a higher risk of obstetric complications, including preeclampsia/eclampsia, venous thromboembolism, intrauterine fetal demise, preterm birth, intrauterine growth restriction, and SCD-related complications, including prepartum and postpartum VOC and ACS. Greater than 50% of patients with SCD have a pain crisis during pregnancy,[54] and 28% will have VOC at the time of delivery.[55] Additionally, approximately 20% of women develop ACS during pregnancy.[56] Furthermore, the maternal mortality rate is 16 times higher and fetal death at delivery is twice as likely in pregnant women with SCD.[57]

Because hydroxyurea may be teratogenic, RBC transfusion is the only disease-modifying therapy for pregnant women with SCD. Transfusion is indicated for women with acute medical or obstetric complications, but conflicting data exist regarding the benefit of regular prophylactic transfusion during pregnancy. Prophylactic transfusion has been proposed to prevent SCD-related and obstetric complications toward the end of pregnancy when they are most frequent. Transfusion may be initiated at 28 weeks' gestation with the goal of maintaining an HbS less than 35% and an Hb of 10 to 11 g/dL.[58] This prophylactic transfusion strategy significantly reduced pain crises and symptomatic anemia but had no effect on pregnancy outcomes in 2 small trials involving 98 women with SCD conducted in the 1980s.[59,60] Recently, prophylactic erythrocytapheresis initiated either in the second or third trimester has been shown in a small single-center retrospective cross-sectional study to be safe and effective in prevention of SCD-related events.[61] Future studies are required to determine if prophylactic transfusions during pregnancy can decrease maternal and perinatal morbidity and mortality associated with SCD. Currently, most obstetricians provide selective transfusion to address specific complications that arise during pregnancy for women with SCD.

Leg Ulcers

Leg ulcers are a common complication of SCD and increase in occurrence with advancing age. By their fourth decade of life, 22% of patients with HbSS and 9% of patients with HbSC will report a history of leg ulcers.[62] Standard treatment of leg ulcers is debridement, wet to dry dressings, topical agents, and prompt treatment of soft tissue infection and/or osteomyelitis.[15] There have been anecdotal reports of transfusion stimulating ulcer healing. Although there are no studies to support chronic transfusion therapy for long-term management, RBC transfusion may be beneficial for patients undergoing surgical debridement, skin grafts, or muscle flaps to promote healing.[63]

Vasoocclusive Crisis

Acute VOC is the most common cause of hospital admissions among patients with SCD. In the Cooperative Study of SCD, mean frequencies of pain episodes for patients with HbSC or HbSβ+, HbSS, and HbSβ° were 0.4, 0.8, and 1.0 episodes per year, respectively.[64] The average hospital stay for VOC is 7.5 days for adults and 4.4 days for children. Treatment of severe VOC requiring hospitalization is pain management with nonsteroidal antiinflammatory drugs and parenteral opioids, intravenous (IV) hydration, and incentive spirometry to minimize the risk of ACS. During acute uncomplicated VOC, mild exacerbation of anemia is common but does not require transfusion. There are no data to support RBC transfusion to manage acute uncomplicated VOC, and transfusion in this setting is associated with a higher risk of RBC alloimmunization.[65] A subset of patients have unusually frequent and severe pain episodes, associated with a poor quality of life. There is empirical evidence that chronic transfusions may reduce acute painful episodes,[11,66] but a concurrent multidisciplinary pain program and periodic assessment for treatment response is required.

Priapism

Priapism affects approximately 35% of boys and men with SCD.[67] Prolonged and recurrent episodes of priapism are associated with tissue necrosis and fibrosis leading to erectile dysfunction. Initial management consists of IV fluids and analgesics; subsequent interventions include penile aspiration and corporal irrigation using α-adrenergic agents. The use of oral pseudoephedrine and low-dose phosphodiesterase type 5 inhibitors has been reported to have prophylactic benefit in SCD-associated priapism, and limited experience suggests hydroxyurea may prevent recurrence.[68] Surgical shunting procedures and penile prosthesis implantation are used when conservative measures fail.[69]

The benefit of RBC transfusion for acute priapism in SCD is controversial. A systematic literature review of patients with SCD-associated priapism reported a mean time to detumescence of 8.0 days in 16 patients who did not receive transfusion compared with 11 days in 26 individuals who received transfusion. The review identified 9 cases of serious neurologic sequelae, including obtundation, seizures, and stroke following transfusion consistent with Association of Sickle cell disease, Priapism, Exchange transfusion, and Neurologic events (ASPEN) syndrome. Most resolved completely but left severe neurologic deficits in some.[70] Given the risk of ASPEN, blood transfusion is not typically recommended to treat acute priapism in patients with SCD. Chronic transfusion therapy is sometimes used to prevent recurrent intermittent priapism, but there is no published evidence of its efficacy. The NHLBI-appointed SCD expert panel recommends against the use of transfusion for the treatment of priapism.[15] **Table 1** summarizes indications for and against transfusion therapy in patients with SCD.

PREVENTION OF COMPLICATIONS
Alloimmunization

RBC alloimmunization is a major complication associated with transfusions in SCD. Alloantibodies to the Rh (primarily C and E) and Kell (typically K) systems compose more than two-thirds of the antibodies detected. The high rate of alloimmunization is multifactorial, but discordance of blood group antigen expression on donor and patient RBCs is likely the major contributing factor. Prevention has focused on prophylactic RBC antigen matching, either limited C, E, K matching or extended antigen matching to include the Duffy, Kidd, and MNS systems (Fy^a, Fy^b, Jk^a, Jk^b, S). Alloimmunization prevalence in patients with SCD ranges from 27% to 75% with ABO-D matching alone, 5% to 14% with limited C, E, and K matching, and 0% to 7% for extended RBC antigen matching (**Table 2**). The rate of alloantibody formation ranges from 1.7 to 3.9 antibodies formed per 100 units transfused with ABO-D matching, 0.26 to 0.50 with limited C, E, K matching, and 0 to 0.10 with extended antigen matching (see **Table 2**).

Limited C-, E-, and K-matched RBCs can reduce alloimmunization (see **Table 2**). Despite consensus in the United States to provide C-, E-, and K-matched RBCs for patients with SCD,[15] this has not been universally practiced.[71,72] Some transfusion services provide extended matched RBCs after patients with SCD have formed one alloantibody, recognizing these patients as "immune responders."[73] In addition to C-, E-, and K-matched RBCs, recruitment of dedicated donors to limit donor exposure for a given patient[74] or providing RBCs from African American donors who are more likely to have similar Jk, Fy, or S antigen status[75] have been alternative strategies used for SCD. In a single-institution study, C-, E-, and K-matched RBCs from African American donors resulted in no cases of anti-K formation and a low rate of anti-Jk, -Fy, and -S antibodies; but Rh immunization remained problematic (**Fig. 1**).[75]

Table 2
Red blood cell antigen matching and alloimmunization

Study	N	Total Units Transfused	Matching	Patients with Alloantibodies (%)	Rate (Alloantibody per 100 Units)
Ambruso et al,[87] 1987	12	492	ABO, D	75	3.5
Rosse et al,[88] 1990	1044	n/a	ABO, D	27	n/a
Vichinsky et al,[89] 1990	107	1711	ABO, D	30	3.9
Aygun et al,[90] 2002	140	3239	ABO, D	37	n/a
Castro et al,[91] 2002	351	8939	ABO, D	29	n/a
Sakhalkar et al,[92] 2005	387	14,263	ABO, D	31	1.7
Vichinsky et al,[93] 2001	61	1830	Limited (C, E, K)	11	0.50
Sakhalkar et al,[92] 2005	113	2354	Limited (C, E, K)	5	0.26
O'Suoji et al,[94] 2013	180	n/a	Limited (C, E, K)	14	n/a
DeBaun et al,[44] 2014	90	3236	Limited (C, E, K)	4.5	0.28
Tahhan et al,[95] 1994	40	608	Extended matching[a]	0	0
Lasalle-Williams et al,[96] 2011	99	6946	Extended matching[b]	7	0.10
Chou et al,[75] 2013	182	44,482	Limited (C, E, K) from African American donors	44	0.33

Abbreviation: n/a, not available.
[a] C/c, E/e, K, Fya, Fyb, S.
[b] C/c, E/e, K, Fya, Jka, Jkb.
Data from Refs.[44,75,87–96]

Inheritance of variant *RHD* and *RHCE* genes encoding amino acid changes in the Rh antigens (D, C, c, E, e) is common in Africans, and its contribution to alloimmunization in patients with SCD despite Rh-matching programs has been increasingly appreciated.[75,76] Many *RH* variants encode partial Rh antigens, and individuals become immunized when exposed to epitopes that their own cells lack.[75,77] *RH* alleles that encode altered D, C, and e antigens often underlie the complex Rh alloantibody and apparent autoantibody specificities found in patients with SCD. Patients form anti-D, -C, and/or -e despite their own RBCs testing positive for those antigens and may represent Rh alloantibodies rather than autoantibodies. These antibodies can be clinically significant, and future transfusions should be with antigen-negative RBCs. This requirement poses significant challenges to transfusion services in providing compatible RBCs to these patients, taking care to avoid additional alloantibody development.

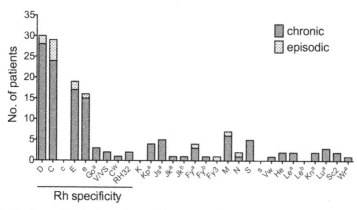

Fig. 1. Antibody specificities in patients with SCD transfused with Rh D-, C-, E-, and K-matched RBCs from African American donors. One hundred forty-six specific antibodies in 123 chronically and 59 episodically transfused patients identified at a single institution over 15 years. (*From* Chou ST, Jackson T, Vege S, et al. High prevalence of red blood cell alloimmunization in sickle cell disease despite transfusion from Rh-matched minority donors. Blood 2013;122(6):1064; with permission. Copyright © the American Society of Hematology.)

Patients with SCD benefit from having an extended RBC antigen phenotype (C/c, E/e, K/k, Fy^a/Fy^b, Jk^a/Jk^b, M/N, S/s, and Le^a/Le^b) completed in the first year of life. Knowledge of RBC antigen status facilitates antibody evaluation and identification of compatible RBC units in patients with a newly formed antibody. RBCs should be matched for C, E, and K antigens at a minimum.[15] Extended antigen-matched RBCs to minimize alloimmunization against Kidd, Duffy, and S antigens is preferable; but finding sufficient RBC units for chronically transfused patients may be challenging for some regions. Overall transfusion cost increases with higher levels of antigen matching, which is prohibitive for many providers. Using molecular blood typing can augment serologic typing and may allow the ability to provide highly antigen-matched products in the future and potentially be cost saving.[78,79]

Altered *RH* alleles in patients with SCD suggest an important emerging role for molecular methods to improve RBC matching in the Rh system.[75,80] Prevention of Rh alloantibody formation in patients with partial antigens is a challenge. Providing antigen-negative RBCs for individuals predicted to exclusively express partial Rh antigens may be performed on an individual case basis, with consideration of their extended RBC antigen profile, alloimmunization history and specificities, and the predicted availability of appropriate donors. For individuals with the relatively common hybrid *RHD*DIIIa-CE(4–7)-D* gene that encodes a partial C antigen, providing C-negative RBCs to those lacking an *RHCE* gene encoding conventional C can minimize anti-C alloimmunization and is consistent with a prophylactic C matching policy.[81] For patients whose *RH* genotypes predict exclusive expression of partial D and/or e antigens, selection of appropriate RBC units is more complex. For example, D-negative units are more likely to be identified among European donors. Providing D-negative RBCs to patients with partial D antigen status may increase alloimmunization risk to other antigens (Fya, Jkb, and S) that are more common in Europeans compared with Africans. As sequencing platforms increasingly improve and become cost-effective, *RH* genotyping can complement serologic testing for both typing and matching donors and patients.

Monitoring and Treatment of Iron Overload

Patients with SCD on chronic or recurrent episodic transfusions are at risk for iron over-load and subsequent liver, endocrine, and/or cardiac dysfunction.[82] Recommendations for monitoring and treatment of iron overload in SCD are largely based on thalassemia literature. Transfusional iron burden should be monitored with serum ferritin levels and liver and cardiac MRI. Liver iron quantification by R2 and R2* MRI techniques correlates well with liver iron content (LIC) determined by liver biopsy.[83] Although less common than comparably transfused patients with thalassemia major, cardiac iron overload occurs in a small proportion of patients with SCD with exceptionally poor control of iron status.[84] In such patients, cardiac T2* MRI can predict the risk of developing heart disease, allowing intensification of therapy.[85] LIC should be measured by R2-MRI every 1 to 2 years while on chronic transfusions and/or if serum ferritin remains greater than 1000 ng/mL. Iron-chelating agents are typically initiated within 1 to 2 years of instituting chronic transfusions, after 10 to 20 cumulative RBC units ($\sim$120 mL/kg), or when LIC is 7 mg/g or greater dry weight.[86] Chelation is titrated to maintain serum ferritin less than 1000 ng/mL and LIC less than 7 mg/g liver dry weight, extrapolated from the thalassemia data.[2]

Iron chelation therapy can maintain a negative iron balance in most compliant patients requiring chronic transfusions. Deferoxamine (25–40 mg/kg/d SQ) and deferasirox (20–40 mg/kg/d by mouth) have been licensed for the treatment of iron overload in SCD, but the safety and efficacy of deferiprone (75–100 mg/kg/d by mouth) has not been established for SCD in the United States. Although deferiprone has been available for patients with SCD outside the United States and Canada since 1995, experience is limited.[2,82]

Unique to SCD, the iron-loading rate of transfusion therapy depends on the modality used (simple vs exchange), the type of exchange (partial manual vs automated), and the target Hb and percentage of HbS.[82] The net iron balance is also influenced by dose and compliance with iron chelation therapy. Patients with severe iron overload may benefit from erythrocytapheresis combined with chelation and by adjusting automated erythrocytapheresis parameters to achieve minimal iron loading. **Tables 3** and **4** provide calculations of transfusion-associated iron accumulation and balance with different transfusion regimens.

Table 3
Calculations of iron accumulation from transfusion

RBC Transfusion Volumes	Amount of Fe Accumulation
1 mL of erythrocytes	Approximately 1 mg of Fe
Fe content of transfused blood	Approximately 0.75 mg/mL (225 mg Fe per 300 mL unit)[a]
Approximately 2 units of RBCs	Approximately 0.5 g of Fe accumulation within the body[b]
10 mL/kg of RBCs	Approximately 7.5 mg Fe/kg
15 mL/kg of RBCs	Approximately 11.3 mg Fe/kg
For chronic transfusions	
10 mL/kg RBCs every 4 weeks	Approximately 0.25 mg/kg/d
15 mL/kg RBCs every 4 weeks	Approximately 0.40 mg/kg/d
15 mL/kg RBCs every 3 weeks	Approximately 0.54 mg/kg/d

Abbreviation: Fe, iron.
  [a] This value assumes a red cell unit hematocrit of 65%.[6]
  [b] Adults normally have approximately 4 to 5 g of total body iron.

Table 4
Iron balance with transfusion regimens

Transfusion Modality	Fe Accumulation (mg/kg/d)[a]	DFX Dosage to Balance Input	DFO Dosage to Balance Input
Simple transfusion			
Target HbS <30%	0.42	20 mg/kg/d	40 mg/kg × 5/wk
Target HbS <50%	0.32	16 mg/kg/d	32 mg/kg × 5/wk
Partial Manual Exchange[b]			
Target HbS <30%	0.36	~18 mg/kg/d	37 mg/kg × 5/wk
Erythrocytapheresis			
Target HbS <30%	0.04–0.08	<5 mg/kg/d	<10 mg/kg × 5/wk
Target HbS <50%	≤0.052	<5 mg/kg/d	<10 mg/kg × 5/wk

Abbreviations: DFO, deferiprone; DFX, deferoxamine; Fe, iron.
[a] These calculations are approximations. The rate of iron accumulation varies within the transfusion modality used based on transfusion volume (10 vs 15 mL/kg), frequency of transfusions (every 3 weeks vs every 4 weeks), phlebotomy volume (partial manual exchange), and after exchange target Hb (erythrocytapheresis).
[b] Fe accumulation approximation for partial manual exchange extrapolated from data calculations from reference.[6]
Adapted from Porter J, Garbowski M. Consequences and management of iron overload in sickle cell disease. Hematology Am Soc Hematol Educ Program 2013;2013:448.

SUMMARY

RBC transfusion is a critical component in the treatment of SCD. Clinicians should be knowledgeable of evidence-based or expert panel–based consensus of transfusion indications and strategies to prevent and manage transfusion-related complications.

REFERENCES

1. Quinn CT. Sickle cell disease in childhood: from newborn screening through transition to adult medical care. Pediatr Clin North Am 2013;60(6):1363–81.

2. Smith-Whitley K, Thompson AA. Indications and complications of transfusions in sickle cell disease. Pediatr Blood Cancer 2012;59(2):358–64.

3. Wahl S, Quirolo KC. Current issues in blood transfusion for sickle cell disease. Curr Opin Pediatr 2009;21(1):15–21.

4. Josephson CD, Su LL, Hillyer KL, et al. Transfusion in the patient with sickle cell disease: a critical review of the literature and transfusion guidelines. Transfus Med Rev 2007;21(2):118–33.

5. Wanko SO, Telen MJ. Transfusion management in sickle cell disease. Hematol Oncol Clin North Am 2005;19(5):803–26, v-vi.

6. Savage WJ, Reddoch S, Wolfe J, et al. Partial manual exchange reduces iron accumulation during chronic red cell transfusions for sickle cell disease. J Pediatr Hematol Oncol 2013;35(6):434–6.

7. Brousse V, Elie C, Benkerrou M, et al. Acute splenic sequestration crisis in sickle cell disease: cohort study of 190 paediatric patients. Br J Haematol 2012;156(5): 643–8.

8. Smith-Whitley K, Zhao H, Hodinka RL, et al. Epidemiology of human parvovirus B19 in children with sickle cell disease. Blood 2004;103(2):422–7.

9. Vichinsky EP, Neumayr LD, Earles AN, et al. Causes and outcomes of the acute chest syndrome in sickle cell disease. National Acute Chest Syndrome Study Group. N Engl J Med 2000;342(25):1855–65.

10. Turner JM, Kaplan JB, Cohen HW, et al. Exchange versus simple transfusion for acute chest syndrome in sickle cell anemia adults. Transfusion 2009;49(5):863–8.

11. Miller ST, Wright E, Abboud M, et al. Impact of chronic transfusion on incidence of pain and acute chest syndrome during the Stroke Prevention Trial (STOP) in sickle-cell anemia. J Pediatr 2001;139(6):785–9.

12. Hankins J, Jeng M, Harris S, et al. Chronic transfusion therapy for children with sickle cell disease and recurrent acute chest syndrome. J Pediatr Hematol Oncol 2005;27(3):158–61.

13. Miller ST. How I treat acute chest syndrome in children with sickle cell disease. Blood 2011;117(20):5297–305.

14. Banerjee S, Owen C, Chopra S. Sickle cell hepatopathy. Hepatology 2001;33(5): 1021–8.

15. Yawn BP, Buchanan GR, Afenyi-Annan AN, et al. Management of sickle cell disease: summary of the 2014 evidence-based report by expert panel members. JAMA 2014;312(10):1033–48.

16. Papafragkakis H, Ona MA, Changela K, et al. Acute liver function decompensation in a patient with sickle cell disease managed with exchange transfusion and endoscopic retrograde cholangiography. Therap Adv Gastroenterol 2014;7(5):217–23.

17. Gardner K, Suddle A, Kane P, et al. How we treat sickle hepatopathy and liver transplantation in adults. Blood 2014;123(15):2302–7.

18. Ahn H, Li CS, Wang W. Sickle cell hepatopathy: clinical presentation, treatment, and outcome in pediatric and adult patients. Pediatr Blood Cancer 2005;45(2): 184–90.

19. Hassell KL, Eckman JR, Lane PA. Acute multiorgan failure syndrome: a potentially catastrophic complication of severe sickle cell pain episodes. Am J Med 1994; 96(2):155–62.

20. Howard J, Malfroy M, Llewelyn C, et al. The Transfusion Alternatives Preoperatively in Sickle Cell Disease (TAPS) study: a randomised, controlled, multicentre clinical trial. Lancet 2013;381(9870):930–8.

21. Vichinsky EP, Haberkern CM, Neumayr L, et al. A comparison of conservative and aggressive transfusion regimens in the perioperative management of sickle cell disease. The Preoperative Transfusion in Sickle Cell Disease Study Group. N Engl J Med 1995;333(4):206–13.

22. Kassim AA, Galadanci NA, Pruthi S, et al. How I treat and manage strokes in sickle cell disease. Blood 2015;125(22):3401–10.

23. Hulbert ML, Scothorn DJ, Panepinto JA, et al. Exchange blood transfusion compared with simple transfusion for first overt stroke is associated with a lower risk of subsequent stroke: a retrospective cohort study of 137 children with sickle cell anemia. J Pediatr 2006;149(5):710–2.

24. Strouse JJ, Lanzkron S, Urrutia V. The epidemiology, evaluation and treatment of stroke in adults with sickle cell disease. Expert Rev Hematol 2011;4(6):597–606.

25. Oyesiku NM, Barrow DL, Eckman JR, et al. Intracranial aneurysms in sickle-cell anemia: clinical features and pathogenesis. J Neurosurg 1991;75(3):356–63.

26. Powars D, Wilson B, Imbus C, et al. The natural history of stroke in sickle cell disease. Am J Med 1978;65(3):461–71.

27. Hulbert ML, McKinstry RC, Lacey JL, et al. Silent cerebral infarcts occur despite regular blood transfusion therapy after first strokes in children with sickle cell disease. Blood 2011;117(3):772–9.

28. Scothorn DJ, Price C, Schwartz D, et al. Risk of recurrent stroke in children with sickle cell disease receiving blood transfusion therapy for at least five years after initial stroke. J Pediatr 2002;140(3):348–54.

29. Ware RE, Helms RW, Investigators SW. Stroke With Transfusions Changing to Hydroxyurea (SWiTCH). Blood 2012;119(17):3925–32.

30. Gyang E, Yeom K, Hoppe C, et al. Effect of chronic red cell transfusion therapy on vasculopathies and silent infarcts in patients with sickle cell disease. Am J Hematol 2011;86(1):104–6.

31. Bishop S, Matheus MG, Abboud MR, et al. Effect of chronic transfusion therapy on progression of neurovascular pathology in pediatric patients with sickle cell anemia. Blood Cells Mol Dis 2011;47(2):125–8.

32. Brousse V, Hertz-Pannier L, Consigny Y, et al. Does regular blood transfusion prevent progression of cerebrovascular lesions in children with sickle cell disease? Ann Hematol 2009;88(8):785–8.

33. Adams RJ, McKie VC, Hsu L, et al. Prevention of a first stroke by transfusions in children with sickle cell anemia and abnormal results on transcranial Doppler ultrasonography. N Engl J Med 1998;339(1):5–11.

34. Enninful-Eghan H, Moore RH, Ichord R, et al. Transcranial Doppler ultrasonography and prophylactic transfusion program is effective in preventing overt stroke in children with sickle cell disease. J Pediatr 2010;157(3):479–84.

35. McCarville MB, Goodin GS, Fortner G, et al. Evaluation of a comprehensive transcranial Doppler screening program for children with sickle cell anemia. Pediatr Blood Cancer 2008;50(4):818–21.

36. McCavit TL, Xuan L, Zhang S, et al. National trends in incidence rates of hospitalization for stroke in children with sickle cell disease. Pediatr Blood Cancer 2013;60(5):823–7.

37. Adams RJ, Brambilla D, Optimizing Primary Stroke Prevention in Sickle Cell Anemia (STOP 2) Trial Investigators. Discontinuing prophylactic transfusions used to prevent stroke in sickle cell disease. N Engl J Med 2005;353(26):2769–78.

38. Abboud MR, Yim E, Musallam KM, et al. Discontinuing prophylactic transfusions increases the risk of silent brain infarction in children with sickle cell disease: data from STOP II. Blood 2011;118(4):894–8.

39. Zimmerman SA, Schultz WH, Burgett S, et al. Hydroxyurea therapy lowers transcranial Doppler flow velocities in children with sickle cell anemia. Blood 2007;110(3):1043–7.

40. Gulbis B, Haberman D, Dufour D, et al. Hydroxyurea for sickle cell disease in children and for prevention of cerebrovascular events: the Belgian experience. Blood 2005;105(7):2685–90.

41. Miller ST, Macklin EA, Pegelow CH, et al. Silent infarction as a risk factor for overt stroke in children with sickle cell anemia: a report from the Cooperative Study of Sickle Cell Disease. J Pediatr 2001;139(3):385–90.

42. Pegelow CH, Macklin EA, Moser FG, et al. Longitudinal changes in brain magnetic resonance imaging findings in children with sickle cell disease. Blood 2002;99(8):3014–8.

43. Schatz J, Brown RT, Pascual JM, et al. Poor school and cognitive functioning with silent cerebral infarcts and sickle cell disease. Neurology 2001;56(8):1109–11.

44. DeBaun MR, Gordon M, McKinstry RC, et al. Controlled trial of transfusions for silent cerebral infarcts in sickle cell anemia. N Engl J Med 2014;371(8):699–710.

45. Kwiatkowski JL, Zimmerman RA, Pollock AN, et al. Silent infarcts in young children with sickle cell disease. Br J Haematol 2009;146(3):300–5.

46. Parent F, Bachir D, Inamo J, et al. A hemodynamic study of pulmonary hypertension in sickle cell disease. N Engl J Med 2011;365(1):44–53.
47. Fonseca GH, Souza R, Salemi VM, et al. Pulmonary hypertension diagnosed by right heart catheterisation in sickle cell disease. Eur Respir J 2012;39(1):112–8.
48. Mehari A, Gladwin MT, Tian X, et al. Mortality in adults with sickle cell disease and pulmonary hypertension. JAMA 2012;307(12):1254–6.
49. Charache S, Terrin ML, Moore RD, et al. Effect of hydroxyurea on the frequency of painful crises in sickle cell anemia. Investigators of the Multicenter Study of Hydroxyurea in Sickle Cell Anemia. N Engl J Med 1995;332(20):1317–22.
50. Voskaridou E, Christoulas D, Bilalis A, et al. The effect of prolonged administration of hydroxyurea on morbidity and mortality in adult patients with sickle cell syndromes: results of a 17-year, single-center trial (LaSHS). Blood 2010;115(12):2354–63.
51. Klings ES, Machado RF, Barst RJ, et al. An official American Thoracic Society clinical practice guideline: diagnosis, risk stratification, and management of pulmonary hypertension of sickle cell disease. Am J Respir Crit Care Med 2014;189(6):727–40.
52. Hayes MM, Vedamurthy A, George G, et al. Pulmonary hypertension in sickle cell disease. Ann Am Thorac Soc 2014;11(9):1488–9.
53. Detterich JA, Kato RM, Rabai M, et al. Chronic transfusion therapy improves but does not normalize systemic and pulmonary vasculopathy in sickle cell disease. Blood 2015;126(6):703–10.
54. Powars DR, Sandhu M, Niland-Weiss J, et al. Pregnancy in sickle cell disease. Obstet Gynecol 1986;67(2):217–28.
55. Alayed N, Kezouh A, Oddy L, et al. Sickle cell disease and pregnancy outcomes: population-based study on 8.8 million births. J Perinat Med 2014;42(4):487–92.
56. Okusanya BO, Oladapo OT. Prophylactic versus selective blood transfusion for sickle cell disease in pregnancy. Cochrane Database Syst Rev 2013;(12):CD010378.
57. Barfield WD, Barradas DT, Manning SE, et al. Sickle cell disease and pregnancy outcomes: women of African descent. Am J Prev Med 2010;38(4 Suppl):S542–9.
58. ACOG Committee on Obstetrics. ACOG practice bulletin No. 78: hemoglobinopathies in pregnancy. Obstet Gynecol 2007;109(1):229–37.
59. Koshy M, Burd L, Wallace D, et al. Prophylactic red-cell transfusions in pregnant patients with sickle cell disease. A randomized cooperative study. N Engl J Med 1988;319(22):1447–52.
60. Koshy M, Burd L, Dorn L, et al. Frequency of pain crisis during pregnancy. Prog Clin Biol Res 1987;240:305–11.
61. Asma S, Kozanoglu I, Tarım E, et al. Prophylactic red blood cell exchange may be beneficial in the management of sickle cell disease in pregnancy. Transfusion 2015;55(1):36–44.
62. Minniti CP, Taylor JG 6th, Hildesheim M, et al. Laboratory and echocardiography markers in sickle cell patients with leg ulcers. Am J Hematol 2011;86(8):705–8.
63. Minniti CP, Kato GJ. How we treat sickle cell patients with leg ulcers. Am J Hematol 2016;91(1):22–30.
64. Platt OS, Thorington BD, Brambilla DJ, et al. Pain in sickle cell disease. Rates and risk factors. N Engl J Med 1991;325(1):11–6.
65. Fasano RM, Booth GS, Miles M, et al. Red blood cell alloimmunization is influenced by recipient inflammatory state at time of transfusion in patients with sickle cell disease. Br J Haematol 2015;168(2):291–300.

66. Styles LA, Vichinsky E. Effects of a long-term transfusion regimen on sickle cell-related illnesses. J Pediatr 1994;125(6 Pt 1):909–11.
67. Olujohungbe AB, Adeyoju A, Yardumian A, et al. A prospective diary study of stuttering priapism in adolescents and young men with sickle cell anemia: report of an international randomized control trial–the priapism in sickle cell study. J Androl 2011;32(4):375–82.
68. Kato GJ. Priapism in sickle-cell disease: a hematologist's perspective. J Sex Med 2012;9(1):70–8.
69. Anele UA, Le BV, Resar LM, et al. How I treat priapism. Blood 2015;125(23):3551–8.
70. Merritt AL, Haiman C, Henderson SO. Myth: blood transfusion is effective for sickle cell anemia-associated priapism. CJEM 2006;8(2):119–22.
71. Afenyi-Annan A, Willis MS, Konrad TR, et al. Blood bank management of sickle cell patients at comprehensive sickle cell centers. Transfusion 2007;47(11):2089–97.
72. Osby M, Shulman IA. Phenotype matching of donor red blood cell units for non-alloimmunized sickle cell disease patients: a survey of 1182 North American laboratories. Arch Pathol Lab Med 2005;129(2):190–3.
73. Karafin MS, Shirey RS, Ness PM, et al. Antigen-matched red blood cell transfusions for patients with sickle cell disease at the Johns Hopkins Hospital. Immunohematology 2012;28(1):3–6.
74. Roberts DO, Covert B, Lindsey T, et al. Directed blood donor program decreases donor exposure for children with sickle cell disease requiring chronic transfusion. Immunohematology 2012;28(1):7–12.
75. Chou ST, Jackson T, Vege S, et al. High prevalence of red blood cell alloimmunization in sickle cell disease despite transfusion from Rh-matched minority donors. Blood 2013;122(6):1062–71.
76. Noizat-Pirenne F, Tournamille C. Relevance of RH variants in transfusion of sickle cell patients. Transfus Clin Biol 2011;18(5–6):527–35.
77. Chou ST, Westhoff CM. The role of molecular immunohematology in sickle cell disease. Transfus Apher Sci 2011;44(1):73–9.
78. Casas J, Friedman DF, Jackson T, et al. Changing practice: red blood cell typing by molecular methods for patients with sickle cell disease. Transfusion 2015;55(6 Pt 2):1388–93.
79. Wilkinson K, Harris S, Gaur P, et al. Molecular blood typing augments serologic testing and allows for enhanced matching of red blood cells for transfusion in patients with sickle cell disease. Transfusion 2012;52(2):381–8.
80. Kappler-Gratias S, Auxerre C, Dubeaux I, et al. Systematic RH genotyping and variant identification in French donors of African origin. Blood Transfus 2014;12(Suppl 1):S264–72.
81. Tournamille C, Meunier-Costes N, Costes B, et al. Partial C antigen in sickle cell disease patients: clinical relevance and prevention of alloimmunization. Transfusion 2010;50(1):13–9.
82. Porter J, Garbowski M. Consequences and management of iron overload in sickle cell disease. Hematol Am Soc Hematol Educ Program 2013;2013:447–56.
83. Wood JC, Enriquez C, Ghugre N, et al. MRI R2 and R2* mapping accurately estimates hepatic iron concentration in transfusion-dependent thalassemia and sickle cell disease patients. Blood 2005;106(4):1460–5.
84. Meloni A, Puliyel M, Pepe A, et al. Cardiac iron overload in sickle-cell disease. Am J Hematol 2014;89(7):678–83.

85. Wood JC. Magnetic resonance imaging measurement of iron overload. Curr Opin Hematol 2007;14(3):183–90.
86. Inati A, Khoriaty E, Musallam KM, et al. Iron chelation therapy for patients with sickle cell disease and iron overload. Am J Hematol 2010;85(10):782–6.
87. Ambruso DR, Githens JH, Alcorn R, et al. Experience with donors matched for minor blood group antigens in patients with sickle cell anemia who are receiving chronic transfusion therapy. Transfusion 1987;27:94–8.
88. Rosse WF, Gallagher D, Kinney TR, et al. Transfusion and alloimmunization in sickle cell disease. The Cooperative Study of Sickle Cell Disease. Blood 1990; 76:1431–7.
89. Vichinsky EP, Earles A, Johnson RA, et al. Alloimmunization in sickle cell anemia and transfusion of racially unmatched blood. N Engl J Med 1990;322:1617–21.
90. Aygun B, Padmanabhan S, Paley C, et al. Clinical significance of RBC alloanti-bodies and autoantibodies in sickle cell patients who received transfusions. Transfusion 2002;42:37–43.
91. Castro O, Sandler SG, Houston-Yu P, et al. Predicting the effect of transfusing only phenotype-matched RBCs to patients with sickle cell disease: theoretical and practical implications. Transfusion 2002;42:684–90.
92. Sakhalkar VS, Roberts K, Hawthorne LM, et al. Allosensitization in patients receiving multiple blood transfusions. Ann N Y Acad Sci 2005;1054:495–9.
93. Vichinsky EP, Luban NL, Wright E, et al. Prospective RBC phenotype matching in a stroke-prevention trial in sickle cell anemia: a multicenter transfusion trial. Transfusion 2001;41:1086–92.
94. O'Suoji C, Liem RI, Mack AK, et al. Alloimmunization in sickle cell anemia in the era of extended red cell typing. Pediatr Blood Cancer 2013;60:1487–91.
95. Tahhan HR, Holbrook CT, Braddy LR, et al. Antigen-matched donor blood in the transfusion management of patients with sickle cell disease. Transfusion 1994;34: 562–9.
96. Lasalle-Williams M, Nuss R, Le T, et al. Extended red blood cell antigen matching for transfusions in sickle cell disease: a review of a 14-year experience from a single center (CME). Transfusion 2011;51:1732–9.

Pathogen Inactivation Technologies
The Advent of Pathogen-Reduced Blood Components to Reduce Blood Safety Risk

Dana V. Devine, PhD[a,b,*], Peter Schubert, PhD[a,c]

KEYWORDS
- Pathogen inactivation • Pathogen reduction technology • Blood safety
- Blood transfusion

KEY POINTS
- Pathogen inactivation technologies (PITs) permit a shift in the blood safety paradigm from reactive to proactive approaches.
- PITs developed for fresh blood components achieve a high degree of pathogen killing as well as inactivation of passenger leukocytes in blood products.
- Although there is some loss of quality using in vitro tests, the clinical performance of treated products is sufficient to warrant acceptance of these first-generation technologies.

SAFETY OF BLOOD PRODUCTS

A major focus in blood transfusion over the past 3 decades has been the improvement of the safety of transfusions with respect to the risk of transfusion-transmitted diseases. Huge amounts of effort and resources have gone into bringing a high level of safety to modern blood products. The approach to increasing the level of blood safety, however, has been reactive. A pathogen is identified and then a test is developed to screen the donor or the blood product for that pathogen. The limitations of a society's financial resources that can be devoted to blood safety in turn limit the success of this strategy. Although large reductions in the risk of transmission of those pathogens for which blood is screened (eg, HIV, hepatitis B, hepatitis C, and West Nile virus) have

Disclosure Statement: The authors have received research funding from Terumo BCT and Macopharma.
[a] Centre for Blood Research, University of British Columbia, 2350 Health Sciences Mall, Vancouver, British Columbia V6T 1Z3, Canada; [b] Canadian Blood Services, 1800 Alta Vista Dr., Ottawa, ON K1G 4J5, Canada; [c] Canadian Blood Services, 2350 Health Sciences Mall, Vancouver, BC V6T1Z3, Canada
* Corresponding author. Centre for Blood Research, University of British Columbia, 2350 Health Sciences Mall, Vancouver, BC V6T1Z3, Canada.
E-mail address: ddevine@pathology.ubc.ca

Hematol Oncol Clin N Am 30 (2016) 609–617
http://dx.doi.org/10.1016/j.hoc.2016.01.005
0889-8588/16/$ – see front matter © 2016 Elsevier Inc. All rights reserved.

been generated, there are other agents that are transmissible in blood for which there currently are not tests readily available or for which implementing testing has not been chosen (eg, *Babesia* and dengue virus).[1] Because the development of blood screening tests is driven by market forces, it is unlikely that new blood screening tests will become available without the demonstration of a high degree of disease burden placed on the recipients of infected blood products. This reactive thinking means that in the months to years between the recognition of the risk of a blood-borne pathogen and the availability of a blood screening test for that agent, recipients are harmed.

This reactive blood safety paradigm was shifted in the plasma proteins industry some time ago. In response to the rise of HIV and the demonstration of its ready transmissibility in fractionated products, especially factor VIII, a multilayered approach to blood safety was developed that not only relied on the screening of donors for known pathogens but also added a series of PITs to the purification and preparation processes for human plasma–derived protein products. These have been highly successful with no transmissions of HIV, hepatitis B, or hepatitis C by fractionated products for approximately 30 years.

For unfractionated blood products, both plasma and cellular, concerns about pathogen transmission remain.[2] Cases of transfusion-transmitted infections and transfusion-associated sepsis still occur,[2] even with the improvement of test sensitivity and concomitant reduction in the window period brought by nucleic acid testing (NAT).[3,4] Detection limits due to low concentration of pathogens at the time of testing, as well as the specter of unknown species not tested for, remain risk factors.

Although the testing of blood for transmissible viruses prior to its release for clinical use has significantly reduced pathogen transmission, not all testing strategies are equally efficacious. An examination of the risk of bacterial transmission in platelet products illustrates the role that the microbial ecology plays in efforts to minimize risk. The contamination of blood products by bacteria most commonly arises from a small number of bacteria that enter the collection bag at the time of donation. With storage at room temperature in a nutrient-rich suspension, the bacteria may multiply many-fold in the days prior to transfusion yet not be at a sufficient concentration to be detected by the gold standard culture methods shortly after preparation. Thus, concerns over potential bacterial contamination of platelet concentrates have limited the shelf life of this product to 5 to 7 days. Other approaches besides testing have also been implemented to increase blood safety. These have included extensive donor screening with improved exclusion criteria, registries of previously deferred donors, prequalification of donors with extended wait periods prior to donation, quarantine of plasma donations until a subsequent donation, donor arm disinfection, and diversion of the first few milliliters of the donation.[5–7]

In an effort to further improve blood safety, lessons from the plasma protein industry began to be applied to component therapy. The advent of PITs brings a profound shift to the overall approach to blood safety. Finally, transfusion medicine can bring a proactive strategy to blood safety rather than remain locked in reactive paradigms. The focus of this review is the current state of PITs for fresh blood components.

CURRENT STATUS OF PATHOGEN INACTIVATION TECHNOLOGIES

The general approach of PITs is to mediate inactivation of pathogens by termination of growth or proliferation rather than an actual reduction (in concentration) of pathogens. Because an organism must be able to reproduce in order to be infectious, this is an effective strategy for preventing transmission of pathogens by blood products. Several pathogen reduction technologies (PRTs) and PITs have been designed that either target the lipid structure of membranes or the RNA/DNA of pathogens that can be used to treat either plasma or cellular products (platelets and red cells). These procedures rely on the illumination of the blood product with UV light in the presence or absence of a photosensitizer. Numerous systems are on the market (**Table 1**) with different approval status in various countries. The available PITs for various blood products are summarized.

Pathogen Inactivation Technologies for Plasma

Solvent/detergent method

Several different approaches have been undertaken to reduce or prevent the transmission of blood-borne pathogens in plasma.[8] The most widespread pathogen inactivation method currently available for plasma involves the combination of a detergent (D) to disturb lipid-enveloped viruses and a nonvolatile solvent (S), in a so-called SD procedure.[9] This approach has proved effective in providing added protection against a wide spectrum of pathogens. Due to their direct negative effects on membranes, SD methods are not applicable to the cellular components of blood but have been adapted for plasma with success and have been licensed and marketed worldwide. The SD method has primarily been applied to pooled plasma, but recently technologies have been developed that allow the treatment of individual plasma units.[10]

Methylene blue

Considerable efforts were directed to the use of photoreactive methylene blue and similar phenothiazine dyes, which have a high affinity for both nucleic acids and the surface structure of viruses. The virucidal activity of methylene blue light treatment has been known for more than a half-century.[11] Some concerns have been expressed about the potential mutagenic effects of methylene blue and its derivatives. Accordingly, an additional filtration step was added to remove the residual dye in the final product with little change in various coagulation parameters.

Amotosalen/UV and riboflavin/UV

Newer technologies that crosslink nucleic acids or generate reactive oxygen species are applicable to plasma. The Intercept system (Cerus, Concord, California) uses the natural compound amotosalen, which intercalates between the nucleotide base pairs of RNA and DNA. The antipathogen activity requires photoactivation by long-wave UV-A light at 320 nm to 400 nm, turning the compound into a reactive intermediate and structural element in the cross-linking of hydrogen-bonded complementary nucleic acid residues.[12] Using a compound absorption device containing activated

Table 1
Pathogen inactivation technologies for fresh blood components

System	Manufacturer	UV (nm)	Photosensitizer	Mechanism of Action
Intercept	Cerus	320–400	Psoralens	Irreversible cross-linking of nucleic acids.
Mirasol	Terumo BCT	280–360	Riboflavin	• Irreversible photo-oxidative damage to nucleic acids • Photolysis of the complex induces guanine oxidation, single strand breaks, and the formation of covalent bonds
Theraflex	MacoPharma	254	None	Nucleic acid damage presumably occurs due to cyclobutyl ring formation

charcoal, unincorporated amotosalen and residual photoproducts are removed from the product prior to use. Potential carryover of remaining amotosalen and its photoproducts in the final blood product required toxicologic evaluation studies that revealed no activity in mutagenicity assays.[13] The Mirasol technology (Terumo BCT, Lakewood, Colorado) works by photoactivation of riboflavin (vitamin B_2) to inactivate pathogens. This compound shares a similarity of structure and mechanism with methylene blue as a photoreactive heterocyclic compound targeting primarily nucleic acids and producing strand cleavage either through an electron transfer process, with oxidation of guanine nucleotide residues and helix fragmentation, or through the production of reactive oxygen intermediates.[14]

From an operational perspective, the Intercept and Mirasol technologies are similar processes. One other difference is the concern with the Intercept process over the unknown long-term safety profile of amotosalen; however, this concern has not been an impediment to regulatory approval. Such concerns are minimal for riboflavin because the compound has an extensive pharmacologic history and has been used in high doses in neonates in the treatment of bilirubinemia.

The treatment of plasma with UV-C alone to inactivate pathogens (Theraflex, Macopharma, Tourcoing, France) is a new development.[15,16]

In summary, methods currently in the marketplace all kill pathogens in plasma albeit with some differences among them as to the degree of kill of specific pathogens. All methods also have the trade-off of increased safety profile for some reduction in the function of the proteins, particularly in the coagulation pathway.[17]

Pathogen Inactivation Technologies for Red Blood Cells

Numerous photosensitizers and alkylating agents have been evaluated for pathogen inactivation of red blood cells (RBCs),[18–20] but many of these caused unacceptable hemolysis or neoantigen formation, precluding commercialization. Candidates currently in late-stage development include the application of a Cerus-developed PIT that is based on an approach similar to Intercept.[21,22]

Pathogen Inactivation Technologies for Platelets

Two PITs, Mirasol and Intercept, discussed previously, are also used for pathogen inactivation of platelet concentrates. There is an additional filtration step in the Intercept procedure that causes a small loss of platelets. For platelets, these PITs are designed to optimize pathogen killing and minimize platelet damage. Using Intercept's amniomethyl trimethylpsoralen (amotosalen [S-59]) requires lower doses of UV, with shorter exposure periods, to achieve virucidal activity for single-stranded DNA or RNA containing viruses.[23] Extensive preclinical toxicologic and pharmacologic studies indicate that there is no evidence of genotoxicity, phototoxicity, or excess carcinogenicity.

For the Mirasol technology, the inactivation principles are the same as for its use in plasma. Like Intercept, the application of the PRT also causes some damage to the platelets, which is expressed as reduced survival and recovery in healthy volunteers with normal platelet counts or as shortened interval to the next transfusion in patients receiving repeated platelet support.[24–26]

Another approach to pathogen inactivation for platelets is under development by Macopharma, which uses UV-C light alone.[27–29] This method uses aggressive agitation of the units during UV exposure to ensure penetration of the UV light throughout the product. Because there are no additives, there is no post-treatment processing required other than placement in a platelet storage container. The inactivation principle is based mainly on UV-C light absorbance by nucleic acids, resulting in the formation of cyclobutane pyrimidine and pyrimidine pyrimidone dimers, which block nucleic acid replication and hence infectivity.

Pathogen Inactivation Technologies for Whole Blood

Ideally, treatment of whole blood prior to component production or without component production is a preferable approach. The development of PITs for whole-blood treatment also is being pursued, although few clinical data are yet available.[30-33] Treatment of whole blood prior to component production offers some significant advantages to blood operators, even though it is likely that the allowable storage time for the RBCs would be shortened.[34]

EFFECT OF PATHOGEN INACTIVATION TECHNOLOGIES ON PATHOGENS

All the PITs currently available or in development effectively inactivate most pathogens.[35] In specific spiking studies, PITs are effective against a variety of pathogens of relevance to blood transfusion.[16,36-41] UV-C alone is less effective on HIV.[42] Because PITs are only effective against pathogens that have nucleic acids, they do not inactivate prions and do not reduce the risk of transmission of variant Creutzfeldt-Jakob disease by blood products (**Table 2**).

EFFECT OF PATHOGEN INACTIVATION TECHNOLOGIES ON THE QUALITY OF BLOOD PRODUCTS

Due the nonspecific nature of PITs, both pathogen and host cell nucleic acids are permanently damaged by treatment. Thus, passenger leukocytes in the components are inactivated, improving the quality of the product. PITs, however, cause some physical damage to the products that may result in a reduction in efficacy compared with untreated products. This negative impact of PITs has not been considered of sufficient severity to outweigh the safety benefit, but it does highlight an area demanding increased effort in the development of improvements to this technology.

Some types of plasma SD treatment cause a significant reduction of anticoagulants α_2-antiplasmin and protein S,[9,43] raising clinical and regulatory concerns over thrombosis risk. Despite some decrease of coagulation factor activity during SD treatment of plasma, clinical trials have repeatedly shown that this decrement does not manifest in increased plasma usage or decreased clinical utility.[44,45]

Both amotosalen and riboflavin PIT systems cause some loss in levels of functional coagulation factors. The pharmacokinetics of fresh frozen plasma photochemically treated with the Cerus system show that the functional activity of coagulation factors was well preserved, with a range of 73% to 98% of control, with no significant differences in von Willebrand factor and its multimers or metalloprotease activity, protein C, protein S, or antithrombin III; and there was no evidence of activation of thrombin, complement, or the contact system, making treated fresh frozen plasma and cryoprecipitate suitable for therapeutic use. Similar findings have been reported for both riboflavin and UV-C inactivation systems.

Numerous in vitro studies report that PITs have some negative effects on the quality of platelet concentrates, including a significant decrease in hypotonic shock response and aggregation, significant acceleration of mitochondrial membrane depolarization and glucose metabolism, and increased P-selectin surface expression indicative of platelet activation.[14,31,46-48] Clinical studies, including those conducted for licensure of these products, show evidence of minor decreases of platelet in vivo survival, but these have not been associated with increased bleeding in patients receiving pathogen-reduced platelets.[24,49-54]

Table 2
Pathogens of concern to transfusion medicine that are inactivated by pathogen reduction technologies

Organism Category	Pathogen	Effectiveness of Inactivation
Protozoa	*Trypanosoma cruzi*	>3 to >6 logs
	Babesia microti	>4 logs
	Malaria sp	
Viruses	HIV	>2.5 to >6.9 logs depending on
	Hepatitis C	PITs or virus testing system
	Hepatitis B	
	Human T-lymphotropic virus-1/II	
	West Nile virus	
	Cytomegalovirus	
	Chikungunya virus	
	Dengue virus	
	Reduced effectiveness against some nonenveloped viruses, such as hepatitis A virus, hepatitis E virus, parvovirus B19	
Bacteria	*Staphylococcus epidermis*	>4 to >7 logs, depending on PIT or
	Staphylococcus aureus	bacterial testing system
	Enterococcus faecalis	Note, bacterial spores may be
	Enterobacter aerogenes	resistant
	Pseudomonas aeruginosa	
	Serratia marcescens	
	Yersinia enterocolitica	
	Klebsiella pneumoniae	
	Escherichia coli	
	Bacillus cereus	
	Boletus aureus	
	Streptococcus agalacticae	
	Streptococcus pyrogenes	
	Enterobacter cloacae	
	Propionibacterium acnes	
	Acinetobacter baumannii	
	Among others	

Although significant data are lacking to assess the effect of PITs on RBCs, it is likely that the application of these technologies will result in a shortening of the storage period to approximately fewer than 42 days. In vitro data show an increase in hemolysis during later storage periods, among other evidence of PIT-induced damage to RBCs.[34]

FUTURE DIRECTIONS

PITs currently have a trade-off between providing reduction of pathogen transmission risk in blood products and reduction of component quality and possible efficacy. Continued research efforts must focus on increasing understanding of the mechanisms by which PITs affect product quality so that strategies can be developed to ameliorate the damage without reducing the pathogen killing efficiency. Dozens of countries have either adopted PIT for the treatment of platelets and/or plasma or are considering doing so. This is a testament to the recognition of the paradigm shift that this technology offers to considerations of blood safety.

REFERENCES

1. Dwyre DM, Fernando LP, Holland PV. Hepatitis B, Hepatitis C and HIV transfusion-transmitted infections in the 21st century. Vox Sang 2011;100:92–8.
2. Vamvakas EC, Blajchman MA. Blood still kills: six strategies to further reduce allogeneic blood transfusion-related mortality. Transfus Med Rev 2010;24:77–124.
3. Iudicone P, Miceli M, Palange M, et al. Hepatitis B virus blood screening: impact of nucleic amplification technology testing implementation on identifying hepatitis B surface antigen non-reactive window period and chronic infections. Vox Sang 2009;96:292–7.
4. Weusten J, Vermeulen M, van Drimmelen H, et al. Refinement of a viral transmission risk model for blood donations in seroconversion window phase screened by nucleic acid testing in different pool sizes and repeat test algorithms. Transfusion 2011;51:203–15.
5. Dodd R, Kurt Roth W, Ashford P, et al. Transfusion medicine and safety. Biologicals 2009;37:62–70.
6. McDonald CP. Bacterial risk reduction by improved donor arm disinfection, diversion and bacterial screening. Transfus Med 2006;16:381–96.
7. Vasconcelos E, Seghatchian J. Bacterial contamination in blood components and preventative strategies: an overview. Transfus Apher Sci 2004;31:155–63.
8. Rock G. A comparison of methods of pathogen inactivation of FFP. Vox Sang 2011;100:169–78.
9. Hellstern P. Solvent/detergent-treated plasma: composition, efficacy, and safety. Curr Opin Hematol 2004;11:346–50.
10. Burnouf T, Radosevich M, El-Ekiaby M, et al. Pathogen reduction technique for fresh-frozen plasma, cryoprecipitate, and plasma fraction minipools prepared in disposable processing bag systems. Transfusion 2011;51:446–7.
11. Seghatchian J, Struff WG, Reichenberg S. Main properties of the THERAFLEX MB-plasma system for pathogen reduction. Transfus Med Hemother 2011;38:55–64.
12. Irsch J, Lin L. Pathogen inactivation of platelet and plasma blood components for transfusion using the INTERCEPT blood system. Transfus Med Hemother 2011;38:19–31.
13. Ciaravino V, McCullough T, Cimino G, et al. Preclinical safety profile of plasma prepared using the INTERCEPT Blood System. Vox Sang 2003;85:171–82.
14. Reikvam H, Marschner S, Apelseth TO, et al. The mirasol pathogen reduction technology system and quality of platelets stored in platelet additive solution. Blood Transfus 2010;8:186–92.
15. Seghatchian J, Walker WH, Reichenberg S. Updates on pathogen inactivation of plasma using Theraflex methylene blue system. Transfus Apher Sci 2008;38:271–80.
16. Seltsam A, Muller TH. UVC irradiation for pathogen reduction of platelet concentrates and plasma. Transfus Med Hemother 2011;38:43–54.
17. Coene J, Devreese K, Sabot B, et al. Paired analysis of plasma proteins and coagulant capacity after treatment with three methods of pathogen reduction. Transfusion 2014;54:1321–31.
18. Wagner SJ. Developing pathogen reduction technologies for RBC suspensions. Vox Sang 2011;100:112–21.
19. Henschler R, Seifried E, Mufti N. Development of the S-303 pathogen inactivation technology for red blood cell concentrates. Transfus Med Hemother 2011;38:33–42.
20. Zavizion B, Pereira M, de Melo Jorge M, et al. Inactivation of protozoan parasites in red blood cells using INACTINE PEN110 chemistry. Transfusion 2004;44:731–8.

21. Cancelas JA, Dumont LJ, Rugg N, et al. Stored red blood cell viability is maintained after treatment with a second-generation S-303 pathogen inactivation process. Transfusion 2011;51:2367–76.

22. Winter KM, Johnson L, Kwok M, et al. Red blood cell in vitro quality and function is maintained after S-303 pathogen inactivation treatment. Transfusion 2014;54: 1798–807.

23. Ciaravi V, McCullough T, Dayan AD. Pharmacokinetic and toxicology assessment of INTERCEPT (S-59 and UVA treated) platelets. Hum Exp Toxicol 2001;20: 533–50.

24. Mirasol Clinical Evaluation Study Group. A randomized controlled clinical trial evaluating the performance and safety of platelets treated with MIRASOL pathogen reduction technology. Transfusion 2010;50:2362–75.

25. Osselaer JC, Messe N, Hervig T, et al. A prospective observational cohort safety study of 5106 platelet transfusions with components prepared with photochemical pathogen inactivation treatment. Transfusion 2008;48:1061–71.

26. van Rhenen D, Gulliksson H, Cazenave JP, et al. Transfusion of pooled buffy coat platelet components prepared with photochemical pathogen inactivation treatment: the euroSPRITE trial. Blood 2003;101:2426–33.

27. Mohr H, Gravemann U, Muller TH. Inactivation of pathogens in single units of therapeutic fresh plasma by irradiation with ultraviolet light. Transfusion 2009;49: 2144–51.

28. Mohr H, Steil L, Gravemann U, et al. A novel approach to pathogen reduction in platelet concentrates using short-wave ultraviolet light. Transfusion 2009;49(12): 2612–24.

29. Thiele T, Pohler P, Kohlmann T, et al. Tolerance of platelet concentrates treated with UVC-light only for pathogen reduction – a phase I clinical trial. Vox Sang 2015;109:44–51.

30. Cancelas JA, Rugg N, Fletcher D, et al. In vivo viability of stored red blood cells derived from riboflavin plus ultraviolet light-treated whole blood. Transfusion 2011;51:1460–8.

31. Marschner S, Goodrich R. Pathogen reduction technology treatment of platelets, plasma and whole blood using riboflavin and UV light. Transfus Med Hemother 2011;38:8–18.

32. Mufti NA, Erickson AC, North AK, et al. Treatment of whole blood (WB) and red blood cells (RBC) with S-303 inactivates pathogens and retains in vitro quality of stored RBC. Biologicals 2010;38:14–9.

33. Fast LD, Nevola M, Tavares J, et al. Treatment of whole blood with riboflavin plus ultraviolet light, an alternative to gamma irradiation in the prevention of transfusion-associated graft-versus-host disease? Transfusion 2013;53:373–81.

34. Schubert P, Culibrk B, Karwal S, et al. Whole blood treated with riboflavin/UV light: quality assessment of all blood components produced by the buffy coat method. Transfusion 2015;55:815–23.

35. Kwon SY, Kim IS, Bae JE, et al. Pathogen inactivation efficacy of Mirasol PRT System and Intercept Blood System for non-leucoreduced platelet-rich plasma-derived platelets suspended in plasma. Vox Sang 2014;107:254–60.

36. Brecher ME, Hay SN. Bacterial contamination of blood components. Clin Microbiol Rev 2005;18:195–204.

37. Singh Y, Sawyer LS, Pinkoski LS, et al. Photochemical treatment of plasma with amotosalen and long-wavelength ultraviolet light inactivates pathogens while retaining coagulation function. Transfusion 2006;46:1168–77.

38. Tonnetti L, Proctor MC, Reddy HL, et al. Evaluation of the Mirasol pathogen reduction technology system against Babesia microti in apheresis platelets and plasma. Transfusion 2010;50:1019–27.
39. Cardo LJ, Salata J, Mendez J, et al. Pathogen inactivation of Trypanosoma cruzi in plasma and platelet concentrates using riboflavin and ultraviolet light. Transfus Apher Sci 2007;37:131–7.
40. Cardo LJ, Rentas FJ, Ketchum L, et al. Pathogen inactivation of Leishmania donovani infantum in plasma and platelet concentrates using riboflavin and ultraviolet light. Vox Sang 2006;90:85–91.
41. Rentas F, Harman R, Gomez C, et al. Inactivation of Orientia tsutsugamushi in red blood cells, plasma, and platelets with riboflavin and light, as demonstrated in an animal model. Transfusion 2007;47:240–7.
42. Schlenke P. Pathogen inactivation technologies for cellular blood products: an update. Transfus Med Hemother 2014;41:309–25.
43. Doyle S, O'Brien P, Murphy K, et al. Coagulation factor content of solvent/detergent plasma compared with fresh frozen plasma. Blood Coagul Fibrinolysis 2003;14:283–7.
44. Hellstern P, Sachse H, Schwinn H, et al. Manufacture and in vitro characterization of a solvent/detergent-treated human plasma. Vox Sang 1992;63:178–85.
45. Piquet Y, Janvier G, Selosse P, et al. Virus inactivation of fresh frozen plasma by a solvent detergent procedure: biological results. Vox Sang 1992;63:251–6.
46. Ostrowski SR, Bochsen L, Windelov NA, et al. Hemostatic function of buffy coat platelets in additive solution treated with pathogen reduction technology. Transfusion 2010;51:344–56.
47. Picker SM, Speer R, Gathof BS. Evaluation of processing characteristics of photochemically treated pooled platelets: target requirements for the INTERCEPT Blood System comply with routine use after process optimization. Transfus Med 2004;14:217–23.
48. Picker SM, Steisel A, Gathof BS. Effects of Mirasol PRT treatment on storage lesion development in plasma-stored apheresis-derived platelets compared to untreated and irradiated units. Transfusion 2008;48:1685–92.
49. AuBuchon JP, Herschel L, Roger J, et al. Efficacy of apheresis platelets treated with riboflavin and ultraviolet light for pathogen reduction. Transfusion 2005;45:1335–41.
50. McCullough J, Vesole DH, Benjamin RJ, et al. Therapeutic efficacy and safety of platelets treated with a photochemical process for pathogen inactivation: the SPRINT Trial. Blood 2004;104:1534–41.
51. Lozano M, Knutson F, Tardivel R, et al. A multi-centre study of therapeutic efficacy and safety of platelet components treated with amotosalen and ultraviolet A pathogen inactivation stored for 6 or 7 d prior to transfusion. Br J Haematol 2011;153:393–401.
52. Osselaer JC, Doyen C, Defoin L, et al. Universal adoption of pathogen inactivation of platelet components: impact on platelet and red blood cell component use. Transfusion 2009;49:1412–22.
53. Sigle JP, Infanti L, Studt JD, et al. Comparison of transfusion efficacy of amotosalen-based pathogen-reduced platelet components and gamma-irradiated platelet components. Transfusion 2013;53:1788–97.
54. Kaiser-Guignard J, Canellini G, Lion N, et al. The clinical and biological impact of new pathogen inactivation technologies on platelet concentrates. Blood Rev 2014;28:235–41.

Transfusion Reactions

William J. Savage, MD, PhD

KEYWORDS

- Transfusion • Reaction • Adverse event • Red blood cell • Platelet • Plasma

KEY POINTS

- Transfusion reactions may be defined by case type, timing, severity, and imputability.
- The differential diagnosis of any untoward clinical event should always consider adverse sequelae of transfusion.
- Fever, dyspnea, hypotension, and urticaria are common manifestations of transfusion reactions.

Transfusion reactions are common occurrences, and clinicians who order or transfuse blood components need to be able to recognize adverse sequelae of transfusion. The differential diagnosis of any untoward clinical event should always consider adverse sequelae of transfusion, even when transfusion occurred weeks earlier. There is no pathognomonic sign or symptom that differentiates a transfusion reaction from other potential medical problems, so vigilance is required during and after transfusion when a patient presents with a change in clinical status. Although transfusion reactions are common, they are uncommonly fatal. The Food and Drug Administration (FDA) receives reports of approximately 40 fatalities attributable to transfusion every year.

Transfusion reactions may be defined by case type, timing, severity, and imputability (the causal relationship of a reaction to transfusion) (**Table 1**). Other classification schemes differentiate reactions by mechanism; for example, immunologic/nonimmunologic, or by type of blood component. This review covers the presentation, mechanisms, and management of transfusion reactions that are commonly encountered, as well as transfusion reactions that can be life-threatening. Approximate risks of selected transfusion reactions are shown in **Fig. 1**.

HEMOLYTIC TRANSFUSION REACTIONS

Hemolytic transfusion reactions are caused by the immune-mediated clearance of transfused red blood cells (RBCs). Immune-mediated hemolysis can be acute or delayed. Hemolytic transfusion reactions are classically thought of as immune-mediated

Disclosure Statement: The author has nothing to disclose.
Transfusion Medicine, Brigham and Women's Hospital, Harvard Medical School, 75 Francis Street, Amory 260, Boston, MA 02115, USA
E-mail address: wjsavage@partners.org

Hematol Oncol Clin N Am 30 (2016) 619–634
http://dx.doi.org/10.1016/j.hoc.2016.01.012
0889-8588/16/$ – see front matter © 2016 Elsevier Inc. All rights reserved.

Table 1
Timing and manifestations of transfusion reactions

Reaction Type	Typical Timing in Relation to Transfusion (Range)	Presenting Signs and Symptoms
Acute hemolytic	During (up to 24 h after)	Fever, chills, dyspnea, hypotension, tachycardia, infusion site pain, back pain, hemoglobinuria, hemoglobinemia, indirect hyperbilirubinemia, renal failure, disseminated intravascular coagulation
Febrile nonhemolytic	During (up to 4 h after)	Fever, chills, rigors
Allergic	During (up to 4 h after)	Urticaria, pruritus, flushing, angioedema, dyspnea, bronchospasm, hypotension, tachycardia, abdominal cramping
Transfusion-associated circulatory overload	Within 2 h (up to 6 h)	Dyspnea, tachycardia, hypertension, headache, jugular venous distention
Septic	During (may be subclinical)	Fever, chills, hypotension, tachycardia, vomiting (may be delayed several hours after transfusion)
Hypotensive	During	Isolated hypotension
Transfusion-related acute lung injury	Within 2 h (up to 6 h)	Dyspnea, hypoxemia, fever, hypotension
Transfusion-associated graft-versus-host disease	8–10 d after (up to 6 wk)	Fever, erythroderma, bloody diarrhea, pancytopenia, liver function abnormalities
Posttransfusion purpura	5–12 d after	Purpura, hemorrhage

Modified from Savage WJ. Transfusion reactions to blood and cell therapy products. In: Hoffman R, Benz E, Silberstein L, et al, editors. Hematology. 7th edition. Philadelphia: Elsevier; in press.

reactions caused by donor RBC antigen incompatibility, but thermal, osmotic, infectious, and mechanical derangements are causes of transfusion-associated hemolysis. Mechanical valves, blood warmers, infusion catheters, and infusion pumps can cause non–alloimmune-mediated hemolytic transfusion reactions. Additionally, free hemoglobin that has leaked into RBC unit supernatant during storage can be passively transfused and can cause hemoglobinuria and hyperbilirubinemia that is not related to acute in vivo hemolysis.[1]

Acute, immune-mediated hemolytic transfusion reactions are those that occur during or immediately after incompatible RBCs are transfused into a patient who already possesses the corresponding antibody. ABO-incompatible RBC transfusion is the prototypical example of an acute hemolytic transfusion reaction. ABO antibodies are spontaneously occurring immunoglobulin (Ig)M and IgG antibodies to A and/or B blood group antigens that are nonself. IgM antibodies efficiently fix complement after binding to ABO-incompatible blood and are responsible for initiating the hemolytic and inflammatory cascades that cause a clinically apparent acute intravascular hemolytic transfusion reaction. Such a reaction could occur, for example, after transfusion of A-type RBCs into an O recipient, who has anti-A. Transfusing as little as 30 mL of incompatible blood can be fatal, and there is a direct relationship between increasing volumes of incompatible blood transfused and mortality.[2]

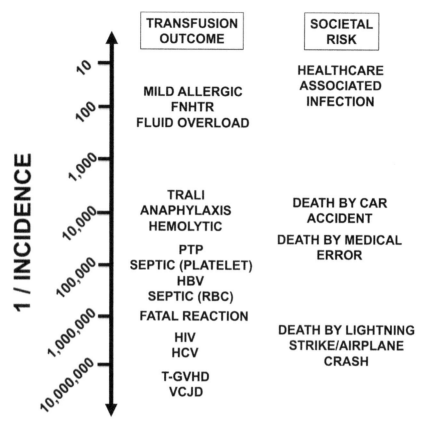

Fig. 1. Approximate risk of select transfusion complications, as compared with select societal risks. VCJD, Variant Creutzfeldt-Jakob disease. (*Modified from* Savage WJ. Transfusion reactions to blood and cell therapy products. In: Hoffman R, Benz E, Silberstein L, et al, editors. Hematology. 7th edition. Philadelphia: Elsevier; in press.)

Acute hemolytic reactions can also occur with incompatible plasma transfusion. Due to platelet inventory constraints, platelet components with plasma incompatible to the recipient are frequently transfused, for example, a group O platelet with anti-A transfused into a group A recipient. Plasma incompatibility (ie, minor ABO incompatibility) can occasionally result in acute hemolytic reactions.[3]

In acute hemolytic transfusion reactions, recipient IgG and/or IgM bound to donor red cells generates anaphylatoxins C3a and C5a, which lead to capillary leak, hypotension, and phagocyte and mast cell activation.[4] Furthermore, the deposition of C3b on the RBC membrane increases extravascular hemolysis. Excessive terminal complement activation results in C5b-9 membrane attack complexes overwhelming complement regulatory factors on the RBC membrane and causes osmotic lysis. Plasma heme also induces renal vasoconstriction through nitric oxide scavenging.[5] In addition to complement components, cytokines also play a role in the clinical syndrome, including fever.[6] For example, interleukin (IL)-1β, IL-6, and tumor necrosis factor (TNF)-α have pyrogenic activity.[7] TNF-α induces tissue factor expression on endothelium while decreasing thrombomodulin, which contributes to disseminated intravascular coagulation (DIC).[8]

An acute intravascular hemolytic transfusion reaction is a medical emergency. Often, the first sign of an immediate hemolytic transfusion reaction is fever, hence the requirement to always stop transfusion and initiate a transfusion workup when fever develops. Other clinical symptoms can include chills, shortness of breath, chest pain, dizziness, flank pain, anxiety, or pain or warmth ascending from the site of infusion. Signs of an acute intravascular hemolytic transfusion reaction are red plasma (hemoglobinemia) and red/dark urine (hemoglobinuria). Acute transfusion reactions can rapidly manifest shock and acute renal failure. Flank pain is common.

Laboratory tests for hemolysis can be useful if there is clinical ambiguity about the type of reaction and for guiding ongoing management of severe hemolytic reactions. Because most ABO-incompatible transfusion reactions are due to errors in safety systems,[9] with an estimated incidence of approximately 1 per 20,000 RBC transfusions,[10,11] an important initial evaluation is confirmation of blood compatibility and determining where an error occurred. There may be a systemic error that could put other patients at risk. Laboratory findings include hemoglobinuria, hemoglobinemia, and a haptoglobin level that is low to undetectable. RBC lysis leads to increased serum lactate dehydrogenase (LDH). If the patient shows no signs of cardiovascular instability and if hemostatic and renal function are unchanged with serial monitoring (for up to a day), serious sequelae are unlikely to develop afterward. The direct antiglobulin test (DAT) may become positive in an immune hemolytic reaction, if tested before all the incompatible RBCs are destroyed.

Initial therapy consists of immediately stopping the transfusion. Treatment interventions follow recommendations for rhabdomyolysis,[12] for which administering alkalinized intravenous fluids is standard. Usually, 0.9% NaCl is infused at 400 mL/h (for adults) to maintain high urine output. Normal saline does not have potassium, which may be problematic in massive hemolysis, but lactated Ringer solution better promotes urine alkalinization.[13] Diuretic use is not clearly beneficial, but a rationale cited is to help clear hemoglobin.[14] Besides managing renal and cardiovascular complications, DIC can occur, so coagulation status should be monitored.

Hyperhemolysis is a type of acute intravascular hemolysis of bystander RBCs that do not express the antigen to which an immune-mediated hemolysis is directed. Hyperhemolysis occurs in the setting of sickle cell disease with transfusion, acute malarial infection, passenger lymphocyte syndrome, paroxysmal nocturnal hemoglobinuria, and select cases of autoimmune hemolytic anemia. Petz and colleagues[15] proposed a term called the "sickle cell hemolytic transfusion reaction syndrome" to describe the constellation of hemolysis, sickle cell pain crisis, reticulocytopenia, severe anemia, RBC transfusion leading to accelerated hemolysis, and lack of a clear serologic reason for hemolysis. Hyperhemolysis is frequently fatal because transfusion exacerbates hemolysis, making anemia worse. Recognition of this syndrome is therefore critical because treatment should shift from transfusion to medical management with erythropoietin, glucocorticoids, and intravenous immunoglobulin (IVIg), which have been used successfully in case series,[16] as well as plasma to RBC exchange transfusion.[17]

DELAYED HEMOLYTIC REACTIONS

The pathogenesis of delayed hemolytic transfusion reactions (DHTR) is similar to that described for an acute hemolytic reaction. However, in DHTRs, the patient develops hemolysis 3 to 10 days after the transfusion as an anamnestic antibody response to a blood antigen previously known to the patient's immune system through transfusion, pregnancy, or hematopoietic stem cell transplantation (HSCT). One study found that half of non-ABO RBC alloantibodies evanesce 6 months after initial detection.[18] If a patient is transfused at another hospital where an antibody screen is negative and a complete transfusion history is not known, incompatible blood can be transfused, setting up a DHTR.

DHTRs are less likely to present as a clinical emergency. Hemoglobinuria and hemoglobinemia can occur but are less pronounced than with an acute intravascular reaction. This may be due to the gradual increase in antibody, and because most DHTRs are due to antibodies not efficient at activating complement. Patients may present with a fever, worsening anemia, and the development of a positive DAT with an eluate demonstrating a new RBC alloantibody. Because these reactions are typically mild in nature, they are usually addressed with supportive care only. In patients with sickle cell disease, DHTRs can precipitate vaso-occlusive crises, autoantibody production, or hyperhemolysis. Thus, it is prudent to take a transfusion history in people with sickle cell disease who present with new complaints.

FEBRILE NONHEMOLYTIC TRANSFUSION REACTIONS

A febrile nonhemolytic transfusion reaction (FNHTR) is suspected when a temperature rise of 1°C to greater than 38°C or more occurs during or after transfusion. In addition to fever, FNHTRs are often associated with rigors and chills. Rigors and chills can also manifest without a concomitant fever, sometimes called an "atypical" or "afebrile" FNHTR. In some cases, temperature increases may be masked by antipyretic premedication. Other causes of isolated fever include acute hemolytic transfusion reactions, septic transfusion reactions, and fever due to underlying disease.

Evidence supports 2 mechanisms of FNHTR: antileukocyte antibodies and a storage lesion of released cytokines. Cytotoxic antibodies having human leukocyte antigen (HLA) specificity, neutrophil specificity, or platelet specificity in the recipient may react against antigens present on transfused donor lymphocytes, granulocytes, or platelets.[19] Similarly, donor plasma may contain antibodies that can react with the cognate cellular antigens in the recipient's blood. Leukocyte-derived cytokines IL-8, IL-1β, and IL-6 accumulate in platelet products, in particular, and induce fever. Higher concentrations of soluble CD40 ligand (CD154) in blood product supernatants have also been associated with FNHTR.[20] Generation of cytokines during storage is directly proportional to the duration of storage.[21,22]

With modern prestorage leukoreduction, the risk of FNHTRs is approximately 1%. Data from pre/post implementation studies show that leukoreduction reduces FNHTRs by 47% to 49% for RBCs and up to 93% for leukoreduction of platelets.[23–25] Risk of FNHTRs increases with storage duration.[26]

The workup of a febrile reaction must be undertaken promptly, because fever may also be the first sign of other, more severe reactions, including acute hemolysis or sepsis. As laboratory testing is being completed, the workup should include bedside patient evaluation. Fever and chills also may be caused by drugs or underlying diseases, or they may be associated with infection or inflammation. Neutropenic fever often complicates the clinical picture in patients undergoing myeloablative chemotherapy, a population likely to undergo multiple RBC and platelet transfusions. Isolated fever may be a sole manifestation of a septic transfusion reaction. It is not routine to identify the specificities of HLA, platelet, or granulocyte antibodies that could cause FNHTRs. Accordingly, the diagnosis of an FNHTR is usually made as a diagnosis of exclusion without isolating an identifiable antibody. Fever from an FNHTR usually responds to antipyretics. Diphenhydramine is not indicated for treatment or prevention or treatment of febrile reactions.

Routine premedication for FNHTRs is unnecessary. Even if a patient has had an FNHTR, most patients do not experience subsequent FNHTRs. Those with a history of clinically significant FNHTRs and those in whom a fever would complicate clinical management (eg, neutropenic patients) may be premedicated with acetaminophen. Those patients with severe reactions despite premedication may require more intensive pharmacotherapy, including corticosteroids, before transfusion. Patients with severe rigors may be treated with meperidine.

Prevention of febrile reactions primarily relies on the use of leukocyte-depleted blood components. Several leukocyte depletion techniques are available. Prestorage leukocyte depletion filters are the most common method used for preventing febrile reactions. They remove up to 4 logs (99.99%) of leukocytes, often lowering the level of white cells in a unit of blood from 10^9 to 10^5. They also are useful for preventing or delaying the onset of HLA alloimmunization and preventing cytomegalovirus (CMV) transmission.[27,28] For these reasons, leukoreduction is universal in many centers. There is a national trend toward universal leukoreduction with approximately 85% of RBC and platelet units leukoreduced.[29] Individuals with a history of recurrent, severe febrile reactions should receive leukocyte-reduced components.

ALLERGIC TRANSFUSION REACTIONS

Allergic transfusion reactions complicate up to 3% of all transfusions.[23,30] Allergic manifestations occur on a spectrum of severity, and they present like other IgE-mediated, immediate hypersensitivity reactions. Signs and symptoms include flushing, urticaria, pruritus, angioedema, hypotension, bronchospasm, stridor, abdominal pain, and emesis. Anaphylaxis is a systemic immediate hypersensitivity reaction, which can be defined as allergic signs and symptoms in skin/mucosa and at least one other organ system (cardiovascular, respiratory, gastrointestinal). Shock is the most ominous manifestation of anaphylaxis, but bronchospasm and upper airway angioedema (eg, hoarseness and stridor) are more common manifestations.

The incidence of allergic transfusion reactions is associated with the amount of plasma in the product. The incidence of reactions to platelets is reduced by approximately two-thirds with concentration or platelet additive solution and approximately 95% with washing.[31,32] Because plasma is associated with these reactions, it is thought that a plasma protein is responsible for many reactions. Examples of IgG or IgE with specificity to IgA, haptoglobin, and C4 have been described, but the incidence of cases with these specificities is rare, and no evidence generalizes these mechanisms to common reactions. There are reports of allergic transfusion reactions to autologous transfusion, suggesting that a storage lesion may be responsible for some reactions.[33] Passive transfer of IgE with allergen exposure in the recipient is a mechanism that has been described for food and antibiotic-mediated allergic transfusion reactions, but these are uncommon.[34–37]

More than 90% of allergic transfusion reactions occur during infusion.[38] When allergic symptoms develop, transfusion should be stopped and the patient given diphenhydramine. The transfusion may resume, but only if the symptoms resolve and the patient feels well. A mild allergic reaction (urticaria and pruritus) during a blood transfusion usually does not progress to a more severe anaphylactic reaction after infusion of additional blood from the same unit. The severity of allergic transfusion reactions is not directly related to volume infused or infusion rate.[39]

Patients who have had mild allergic reactions may continue to receive routine units. Washed RBCs or plasma-reduced platelets can be used to prevent severe, recurrent reactions; however, washing cellular products compromises component quality and reduces posttransfusion corrected count increment by approximately 20% for plate-lets.[40] Washing RBCs leads to accelerated in vitro hemolysis within 24 hours, especially with older methods.[41]

There is no evidence that antihistamine premedication prevents allergic transfusion reactions, although antihistamines do mitigate symptoms when they occur. Studies in healthy volunteers support a synergistic role for treating histamine-mediated reactions with both H1 and H2 receptor antagonists, for example, diphenhydramine and raniti-dine, respectively. Corticosteroids, provided in advance of a transfusion, also may be useful in patients with serious recurrent reactions. Nonsedating antihistamines, for example, cetirizine, have not been extensively studied in the context of allergic trans-fusion reactions, but there is strong mechanistic rationale that they should alleviate symptoms.

Most anaphylactic transfusion reactions are idiopathic. Case reports describe mod-erate or severe anaphylactic reactions in patients who are severely IgA deficient (<0.05 mg/dL) and have anti-IgA antibodies. The generalizability of this mechanism is low. Most cases of fatal anaphylaxis are not related to IgA deficiency, and most peo-ple with severe IgA deficiency tolerate transfusions well.[42] Thus, patients with inci-dental IgA deficiency may receive routine blood components, and IgA/anti-IgA testing should be reserved for patients with anaphylactic reactions. Quantitative haptoglobin can also be considered as a screening test, as rare cases of haptoglobin deficiency are associated with anaphylactic reactions.[43]

HYPOTENSIVE TRANSFUSION REACTION

A less recognized, but severe acute transfusion reaction is isolated hypotension during or immediately following a blood product infusion. For adults, the definition includes a drop in systolic blood pressure of more than 30 mm Hg to below 80 mm Hg. Most commonly, hypotension occurs within minutes of the start of the transfusion and resolves quickly after the transfusion is stopped. Two-thirds of cases involve surgical or critically ill patients with an overall incidence of 1 in 10,000 units transfused.[44] The pathogenesis of this syndrome appears to be related to the activa-tion of the contact pathway (prekallikrein converting to kallikrein) induced in plasma by the negatively charged surface of some leukoreduction filters. Kallikrein activation stimulates the conversion of high-molecular-weight kininogen to bradykinin. The syn-drome is often more severe in patients already taking angiotensin-converting enzyme inhibitors, which doubles the half-life of bradykinin degradation product des-Arg9-BK.[45] Two surgical settings that may pose increased risk of hypotensive reactions include (1) procedures involving the prostate, because another kallikrein gene family member, hK2, can generate bradykinin, and (2) cardiac bypass surgery, because the pulmonary vasculature is an important site for kinin metabolism.

INFECTIOUS COMPLICATIONS OF TRANSFUSION

Bacterial contamination of stored blood poses grave risk to the recipient. Bacteria may enter the blood collection bag with venipuncture during collection, but other routes of contamination include component preparation and occult bacteremia in the blood donor. Platelet concentrates, stored at room temperature, have the highest risk of bacterial contamination. Many reports describe fatal septic transfusion reactions due to platelets containing a variety of species, usually skin flora.[46] Bacteria that grow well at refrigerated blood bank temperatures (1°C to 6°C), including *Pseudo-monas, Yersinia, Enterobacter,* and *Flavobacterium,* are organisms commonly associ-ated with a contaminated unit of RBCs.[47] Units of blood that are contaminated need not be discolored, malodorous, or clotted: blood bags are gas permeable and blood components are cellular suspensions, just as bacteria are in a contaminated unit.

Patients who receive a unit of contaminated blood may develop fever, rigors, skin flushing, abdominal cramps, myalgias, DIC, renal failure, and shock. Just as gram-negative bacteria present more severely with clinical sepsis, gram-negative blood component contamination usually presents more severely than gram-positive contamination. Reactions may be immediate, or there may be a delay of several hours before the symptoms become apparent, especially with gram-positive bacteria. Transfusion of gram-positive bacteria may not be distinguishable from an FNHTR. Shock in a septic transfusion reaction is attributable to endotoxin produced by gram-negative bacteria. Septic transfusions differ from acute hemolytic reactions most notably by the absence of characteristic hemoglobinuria and hemoglobinemia.

When a patient who appeared well suddenly develops rigors, fever, and/or shock during a transfusion, an infected component should be considered. Blood infusion should be stopped the moment a transfusion reaction is suspected, and appropriate samples should be sent to the blood bank for a DAT, hemolysis check, and Gram stain/bacterial culture. It is also important to consider a bacterially contaminated blood component when a previously asymptomatic patient presents with signs of bacteremia several hours after a transfusion is completed.

Because of the decrease in viral transmission by blood transfusion over the past 3 decades, septic transfusion reactions now account for a significant portion of the transfusion-related infections in the United States. Data from the Bacterial Contamination of Blood study showed that from 1998 to 2000, the rate of transfusion-transmitted bacteremia was approximately 1 per 100,000 for platelets and approximately 1 per 5,000,000 for RBC units.[48] Approximately 1 in 5 septic platelet transfusions and 1 in 2 septic red cell transfusions are fatal. To decrease the likelihood of a septic unit of platelets being transfused, the expiration date of units of platelet concentrate has been limited to a 5-day outdate. To further reduce the risk for bacterial transmission through platelet transfusion, platelet concentrates must be tested for bacterial contamination.

Nonbacterial microbial transmission through transfusion does not lead to acute reactions. Rather, subacute infectious syndromes present days to months after transfusion. Viruses that are current threats to transfusion safety include human immunodeficiency virus (HIV), hepatitis A virus, hepatitis B virus (HBV), hepatitis C virus (HCV), human T lymphotropic virus, West Nile virus (WNV), dengue, parvovirus, Zika virus and chikungunya. CMV viremia occurs in approximately 1% of transfused CMV-negative HSCT patients.[49] Blood donors with viral syndromes at the time of donation are excluded from the blood supply as a precaution to minimize the chance that other viruses could be transferred to patients, many of whom are immunocompromised and at risk of more severe viral infectious sequelae. Of the parasites known to be transmitted through blood transfusion, *Babesia microti* has the highest incidence, especially in the Northeast and upper Midwest of the United States, with 160 cases reported through 2009.[50] *Babesia* is also the leading cause of transfusion-transmitted infectious mortality.[51] Other parasites transmitted through blood transfusion include *Plasmodium*, *Trypanosoma cruzi*, *Anaplasma*, *Rickettsia*, and *Leishmania*. As with bacteremia, it is important to always consider transfusion as an infectious source in patients with a transfusion history. With the advent of nucleic acid screening, the risks of viral transmission have decreased dramatically, but the risks cannot be eliminated. The current risk of HIV and HCV from transfusion is less than 1 in 2,000,000; HBV has a slightly higher risk of approximately 1 in 300,000 because of a longer window period.[52,53]

Emerging threats to blood safety are ever present. After identification in the United States in 1999, WNV emerged as a transfusion-transmissible infection in 2002, leading initially to 23 confirmed infections and likely hundreds of undocumented cases.[54,55] Nucleic acid testing is now standard for WNV, reducing the residual risk to less than 1 case nationally per year.[56] Dengue, and likely chikungunya and Zika virus as well, can be transmitted through blood transfusion,[57,58] and prevalence is increasing in North America.[59,60] Strategies to reduce the risk of emerging threats in blood products is an active area of investigation, centered largely around pathogen-reduction techniques involving UV irradiation with or without chemical adjuncts, for example, riboflavin or amotosalen.[61,62]

TRANSFUSION-RELATED ACUTE LUNG INJURY

Transfusion-related acute lung injury (TRALI) is the leading cause of transfusion-related death reported to the FDA. For the period of 2010 to 2014, 41% (72 of 176) of reported fatalities to the FDA were due to TRALI.[51] Currently, approximately 1 in 10,000 transfusions is complicated by TRALI.[63] Symptoms of TRALI range from mild dyspnea to severe noncardiogenic pulmonary edema, often accompanied by chills, fever, and hypotension. Patients require oxygen support, and many require mechanical ventilation. TRALI by definition develops within 6 hours of starting a transfusion, but typically reactions occur within 2 hours.[64] Because the pulmonary edema is noncardiogenic, there is classically no elevation in cardiopulmonary pressures.

It is postulated that TRALI consists of a 2-hit event, the first hit being an underlying clinical condition that leads to the sequestration and priming of neutrophils in the lung tissue, and the second being the transfusion of blood products containing anti-HLA or anti-human neutrophil antigen (HNA) antibodies that activate the neutrophils in the lung parenchyma, leading to edema.[65,66] Previously pregnant women make anti-neutrophil and anti-HLA antibodies, and blood donations from this population are the primary source of anti-neutrophil and anti-HLA antibodies.[67] Removal of female donors from the plasma component pool has resulted in a reduction in TRALI by approximately half.[63,68] Other, antibody-independent mechanisms of TRALI have been described. It been reported that aged blood products may accumulate bioactive lipids and soluble mediators, such as CD40 L, that hamper the chemokine scavenging ability of erythrocytes, and this may represent a second hit in the 2-hit model.[69] Lysophosphatidyl choline accumulation during storage is another neutrophil priming substance that is transfused.[70]

Because TRALI is hard to distinguish from fluid overload without central cardiovascular pressure measurements, it is not straightforward to diagnose. HLA/neutrophil antigen-antibody reactions are usually donor specific and should not recur with a unit from a different donor. Treatment is supportive. Glucocorticoids and diuretics have not been established to help, although a positive fluid balance is a risk factor for TRALI.[63] Donors who are clearly implicated in TRALI reactions should be permanently deferred from blood donation. Hence, reporting of these reactions to the blood bank is important so that implicated donors can be identified and tested.

TRANSFUSION-ASSOCIATED CIRCULATORY OVERLOAD

Transfusion-associated circulatory overload (TACO) results from hydrostatic transudate accumulation in the lungs and should be considered in patients who, during blood infusion, develop sudden onset of dyspnea, jugular venous distention, tachycardia, congestive heart failure, or other signs of fluid overload. Unless there is severe hemorrhage or life-threatening shock, blood should not be infused rapidly. Patients with compromised cardiopulmonary status may not tolerate acute blood volume expansion and may develop right-sided or left-sided heart failure. This is especially true for infants, the elderly, and people with renal and heart failure.

TACO is a transfusion reaction and must be reported to the blood bank. Prospective studies indicate that TACO is vastly underreported. The estimated incidence is approximately 1 per 100 transfusions.[71,72] If TACO is suspected, the transfusion should be stopped and the patient's blood volume reduced by diuretics. If there is significant concern that the patient may not tolerate infusion of a full unit within the 4-hour period allotted for infusion, the blood bank may divide the product into aliquots for separate transfusions, spaced out in time. As a general guide, infusions in adults should occur at less than 3 mL/kg per hour. The rate should be lowered to 1 mL/kg per hour or infusion for the full 4 hours before product expiration for patients at risk for fluid overload. For a blood component of 300 mL with a typical 4-hour expiration, a 75-kg adult would receive the component at 1 mL/kg per hour if transfused over 4 hours. Diuretics may be given to patients with compromised cardiopulmonary status before transfusion. Diagnostically, respiratory improvement with diuresis suggests TACO.

The initial stages of transfusion-induced hypervolemia may be difficult to distinguish from hemolytic transfusion reaction, FNHTR, allergic reaction, or TRALI. The absence of hemoglobinuria and hemoglobinemia and the absence of a positive posttransfusion DAT result distinguish the reaction from one caused by immune hemolysis. Likewise, the absence of fever, chills, or urticaria should help distinguish TACO from the febrile or allergic types of reactions. The clinical use of laboratory testing, such as N-terminal pro-brain natriuretic peptide (NT-proBNP), may aid in the diagnosis; when NT-proBNP is at least 50% higher after transfusion than pretransfusion levels, NT-proBNP is sensitive and specific for TACO and makes other diagnoses in the differential less likely.[73–75] TRALI is less likely when NT-proBNP is elevated.

TRANSFUSION-ASSOCIATED GRAFT-VERSUS-HOST DISEASE

Transfusion-associated graft-versus-host disease (t-GVHD) occurs when immunologically competent lymphocytes are introduced into a host who cannot inactivate the donor lymphocytes. The immunocompetent donor lymphocytes engraft, host HLA antigen is presented to donor lymphocytes, and the activated lymphocytes attack host tissues. t-GVHD occurs after transfusion of nonirradiated cellular blood components. t-GVHD has a much higher fatality rate than HSCT-related GVHD because the donor lymphocytes produce recipient bone marrow aplasia in addition to typical liver, gut, and skin manifestations of acute GVHD. In GVHD after bone marrow transplantation, the bone marrow is of donor origin, and bone marrow aplasia does not occur.

t-GVHD is fatal in more than 90% of cases, primarily because of aplasia of the recipient's bone marrow. It often occurs 8 to 10 days after transfusion with marked pancytopenia, as well as gut, skin, and liver GVHD.[76] The signs and symptoms include nausea, vomiting, anorexia, fever, diarrhea, liver dysfunction, and erythroderma.[77] Patients often die of infection and hemorrhage within 3 to 4 weeks. There is no effective treatment, with the possible exception of bone marrow transplantation, if posttransfusion GVHD is recognized early and a suitable donor can be found in a short time.

Reports have shown that haploidentical directed donor units of blood may produce fatal posttransfusion GVHD even in immunocompetent recipients, when donor and recipient share HLA types.[78] The use of irradiated blood (2500 cGy) is thus recommended in clinical situations in which posttransfusion GVHD is considered possible, such as when patients receive directed blood transfusions from their relatives. Leukocyte-reduction filters should not be used as prophylaxis against GVHD, because the number of leukocytes needed to produce t-GVHD is not known. Case reports of fatal GVHD in patients who received leukoreduced, but not irradiated, blood have been published.[79,80] GVHD continues to be a rare, but extremely serious, complication of blood transfusion. From 2010 to 2014, 2 fatalities from transfusion-associated GVHD were reported to the FDA.[51] Irradiation of RBCs causes membrane damage, permitting slow leakage of potassium and hemoglobin extracellularly.[41] Nevertheless, rather than track which patients need irradiated blood, some centers provide universal irradiation of RBC components without adverse sequelae.

POSTTRANSFUSION PURPURA

Occurring in roughly 1 in 100,000 transfusions, posttransfusion purpura (PTP) is a rare, self-limited thrombocytopenia occurring 5 to 10 days after transfusion in patients lacking a specific platelet antigen, usually HPA-1a (GPIIIa, CD61).[81] These patients typically have a history of sensitization with prior transfusions or pregnancies. Indeed, approximately 85% of cases occur in women.[82] After reexposure with transfusion, patients can develop potent antibodies against the platelet-specific antigen that they are lacking but which is present on donor platelets. These platelet antibodies often have a high titer and can fix complement, destroying the patient's own platelets through indiscriminant adsorption of the antigen or immune complexes on their own platelets. The thrombocytopenia can be marked with a platelet count falling below 10,000/μL.

The onset is sudden, although self-limited, and usually resolves in 2 weeks. This severe thrombocytopenia can help distinguish PTP from heparin-induced thrombocytopenia, which can also be considered in the differential diagnosis when thrombocytopenia develops 5 to 10 days after combined heparin exposure and blood transfusion, for example, major surgery.[83] PTP can be considered if platelet refractoriness continues despite transfusion of HLA-matched platelets. IVIg appears to be an effective treatment, although plasma exchange, steroids, and splenectomy also may be useful.[84–86] Patients with acute bleeding and needing platelet support should receive platelets without the platelet-specific antigen, if possible. If random donor platelets are given, patients can develop severe inflammatory reactions.

AIR EMBOLI

Air may be infused into patients by the roller pumps contained in various transfusion devices, especially apheresis machines and intraoperative salvage machines. All such devices currently use air-in-line sensors. Use and removal of central lines also may pose a risk for air embolism. Patients who receive large volumes of air intravenously experience acute cardiopulmonary insufficiency. The air tends to lodge in the right ventricle, preventing blood from entering the pulmonary circulation. Acute cyanosis, pain, cough, shock, and arrhythmia may occur, and death may result unless immediate action is taken. The patient should be placed head-down on the left side; this may displace the air bubble from the pulmonary valve. Trendelenburg position is also acceptable. High-flow 100% oxygen should be administered. Vascular air aspiration, cardiac compressions, hyperbaric oxygen, and cardiovascular support with dobutamine are other options.[87]

NATIONAL HEALTHCARE SAFETY NETWORK

The National Healthcare Safety Network (NHSN) is a national program of combined governmental and private sector agencies that evaluates and tracks transfusion adverse effects using a protocol called the Hemovigilance Module. Similar programs exist in other countries, including the United Kingdom (Serious Hazards of Transfusion, SHOT), the Netherlands (Transfusion and Transplantation Related Incidents in Patients, TRIP), and Canada (Transfusion Transmitted Injuries Surveillance System, TTISS). Hemovigilance systems in other countries have established efficacy of safety interventions, for example, reduction in TRALI using male-only plasma donors. These systems can also identify emerging threats to transfusion safety, especially when events are uncommon and are detectable only when large numbers of outcomes are evaluated in aggregate.

The Hemovigilance Module provides standard criteria and definitions to participating facilities to report adverse events related to blood transfusion that will result in aggregate data suitable for trend analyses and benchmarking (http://www.cdc.gov/nhsn/PDFs/Biovigilance/BV-HV-protocol-current.pdf).

SUMMARY

Blood and blood component transfusion has inherent risks. Immediate and severe reactions can be straightforward to detect, but vigilance is needed to recognize delayed reactions or reactions presenting with nonspecific signs and symptoms, such as fever or dyspnea. Although the incidence of many adverse sequelae from transfusion is decreasing, there are always emerging threats to transfusion safety. Reporting any suspected reaction to the blood bank is critical for many reasons, including that there may be donors or related components yet to be transfused that need to be removed from the blood supply.

REFERENCES

1. L'Acqua C, Bandyopadhyay S, Francis RO, et al. Red blood cell transfusion is associated with increased hemolysis and an acute phase response in a subset of critically ill children. Am J Hematol 2015;90(10):915–20.
2. Janatpour KA, Kalmin ND, Jensen HM, et al. Clinical outcomes of ABO-incompatible RBC transfusions. Am J Clin Pathol 2008;129:276–81.
3. Josephson CD, Castillejo MI, Grima K, et al. ABO-mismatched platelet transfusions: strategies to mitigate patient exposure to naturally occurring hemolytic antibodies. Transfus Apher Sci 2010;42:83–8.
4. Stowell SR, Winkler AM, Maier CL, et al. Initiation and regulation of complement during hemolytic transfusion reactions. Clin Dev Immunol 2012;2012:307093.
5. Donadee C, Raat NJ, Kanias T, et al. Nitric oxide scavenging by red blood cell microparticles and cell-free hemoglobin as a mechanism for the red cell storage lesion. Circulation 2011;124:465–76.
6. Hod EA, Cadwell CM, Liepkalns JS, et al. Cytokine storm in a mouse model of IgG-mediated hemolytic transfusion reactions. Blood 2008;112:891–4.
7. Muylle L, Joos M, Wouters E, et al. Increased tumor necrosis factor alpha (TNF alpha), interleukin 1, and interleukin 6 (IL-6) levels in the plasma of stored platelet concentrates: relationship between TNF alpha and IL-6 levels and febrile transfusion reactions. Transfusion 1993;33:195–9.
8. Davenport RD, Polak TJ, Kunkel SL. White cell-associated procoagulant activity induced by ABO incompatibility. Transfusion 1994;34:943–9.
9. Bolton-Maggs PH. Bullet points from SHOT: key messages and recommendations from the Annual SHOT Report 2013. Transfus Med 2014;24:197–203.
10. Linden JV, Wagner K, Voytovich AE, et al. Transfusion errors in New York State: an analysis of 10 years' experience. Transfusion 2000;40:1207–13.

11. Kleinman S, Chan P, Robillard P. Risks associated with transfusion of cellular blood components in Canada. Transfus Med Rev 2003;17:120–62.
12. Zimmerman JL, Shen MC. Rhabdomyolysis. Chest 2013;144:1058–65.
13. Cho YS, Lim H, Kim SH. Comparison of lactated Ringer's solution and 0.9% saline in the treatment of rhabdomyolysis induced by doxylamine intoxication. Emerg Med J 2007;24:276–80.
14. Parekh R, Care DA, Tainter CR. Rhabdomyolysis: advances in diagnosis and treatment. Emerg Med Pract 2012;14:1–15 [quiz: 15].
15. Petz LD, Calhoun L, Shulman IA, et al. The sickle cell hemolytic transfusion reaction syndrome. Transfusion 1997;37:382–92.
16. Danaee A, Inusa B, Howard J, et al. Hyperhemolysis in patients with hemoglobinopathies: a single-center experience and review of the literature. Transfus Med Rev 2015;29(4):220–30.
17. Uhlmann EJ, Shenoy S, Goodnough LT. Successful treatment of recurrent hyperhemolysis syndrome with immunosuppression and plasma-to-red blood cell exchange transfusion. Transfusion 2014;54:384–8.
18. Tormey CA, Stack G. The persistence and evanescence of blood group alloantibodies in men. Transfusion 2009;49:505–12.
19. Brubaker DB. Clinical significance of white cell antibodies in febrile nonhemolytic transfusion reactions. Transfusion 1990;30:733–7.
20. Blumberg N, Gettings KF, Turner C, et al. An association of soluble CD40 ligand (CD154) with adverse reactions to platelet transfusions. Transfusion 2006;46:1813–21.
21. Kaufman J, Spinelli SL, Schultz E, et al. Release of biologically active CD154 during collection and storage of platelet concentrates prepared for transfusion. J Thromb Haemost 2007;5:788–96.
22. Shanwell A, Falker C, Gulliksson H. Storage of platelets in additive solutions: the effects of magnesium and potassium on the release of RANTES, beta-thromboglobulin, platelet factor 4 and interleukin-7, during storage. Vox Sang 2003;85:206–12.
23. Heddle NM, Blajchman MA, Meyer RM, et al. A randomized controlled trial comparing the frequency of acute reactions to plasma-removed platelets and prestorage WBC-reduced platelets. Transfusion 2002;42:556–66.
24. King KE, Shirey RS, Thoman SK, et al. Universal leukoreduction decreases the incidence of febrile nonhemolytic transfusion reactions to RBCs. Transfusion 2004;44:25–9.
25. Paglino JC, Pomper GJ, Fisch GS, et al. Reduction of febrile but not allergic reactions to RBCs and platelets after conversion to universal prestorage leukoreduction. Transfusion 2004;44:16–24.
26. Sarkodee-Adoo CB, Kendall JM, Sridhara R, et al. The relationship between the duration of platelet storage and the development of transfusion reactions. Transfusion 1998;38:229–35.
27. Leukocyte reduction and ultraviolet B irradiation of platelets to prevent alloimmunization and refractoriness to platelet transfusions. The Trial to Reduce Alloimmunization to Platelets Study Group. N Engl J Med 1997;337:1861–9.
28. Bowden RA, Slichter SJ, Sayers MH, et al. Use of leukocyte-depleted platelets and cytomegalovirus-seronegative red blood cells for prevention of primary cytomegalovirus infection after marrow transplant. Blood 1991;78:246–50.
29. National Blood Collection and Utilization Survey Report. 2012. Available at: http://www.hhs.gov/ash/bloodsafety/nbcus/. Accessed August 23, 2015.

30. Slichter SJ, Kaufman RM, Assmann SF, et al. Dose of prophylactic platelet transfusions and prevention of hemorrhage. N Engl J Med 2010;362:600–13.
31. Tobian AA, Savage WJ, Tisch DJ, et al. Prevention of allergic transfusion reactions to platelets and red blood cells through plasma reduction. Transfusion 2011;51:1676–83.
32. Tobian AA, Fuller AK, Uglik K, et al. The impact of platelet additive solution apheresis platelets on allergic transfusion reactions and corrected count increment (CME). Transfusion 2014;54(6):1523–9.
33. Domen RE, Hoeltge GA. Allergic transfusion reactions: an evaluation of 273 consecutive reactions. Arch Pathol Lab Med 2003;127:316–20.
34. Ponnampalam A, Growe G, Loftus P, et al. Acquired peanut hypersensitivity following platelet transfusion. Transfus Med 2014;24(6):426–7.
35. Arnold DM, Blajchman MA, Ditomasso J, et al. Passive transfer of peanut hypersensitivity by fresh frozen plasma. Arch Intern Med 2007;167:853–4.
36. Poisson JL, Riedo FX, Aubuchon JP. Acquired peanut hypersensitivity after transfusion. Transfusion 2014;54:256–7.
37. Branch DR, Gifford H. Allergic reaction to transfused cephalothin antibody. JAMA 1979;241:495–6.
38. Savage WJ, Hamilton RG, Tobian AA, et al. Defining risk factors and presentations of allergic reactions to platelet transfusion. J Allergy Clin Immunol 2014; 133:1772–5.e9.
39. Savage WJ, Tobian AA, Savage JH, et al. Transfusion and component characteristics are not associated with allergic transfusion reactions to apheresis platelets. Transfusion 2015;55:296–300.
40. Karafin M, Fuller AK, Savage WJ, et al. The impact of apheresis platelet manipulation on corrected count increment. Transfusion 2012;52(6):1221–7.
41. O'Leary MF, Szklarski P, Klein TM, et al. Hemolysis of red blood cells after cell washing with different automated technologies: clinical implications in a neonatal cardiac surgery population. Transfusion 2011;51:955–60.
42. Sandler SG, Eder AF, Goldman M, et al. The entity of immunoglobulin A-related anaphylactic transfusion reactions is not evidence based. Transfusion 2015; 55(1):199–204.
43. Shimada E, Tadokoro K, Watanabe Y, et al. Anaphylactic transfusion reactions in haptoglobin-deficient patients with IgE and IgG haptoglobin antibodies. Transfusion 2002;42:766–73.
44. Pagano MB, Ness PM, Chajewski OS, et al. Hypotensive transfusion reactions in the era of prestorage leukoreduction. Transfusion 2015;55:1668–74.
45. Cyr M, Hume HA, Champagne M, et al. Anomaly of the des-Arg9-bradykinin metabolism associated with severe hypotensive reactions during blood transfusions: a preliminary study. Transfusion 1999;39:1084–8.
46. Yomtovian RA, Palavecino EL, Dysktra AH, et al. Evolution of surveillance methods for detection of bacterial contamination of platelets in a university hospital, 1991 through 2004. Transfusion 2006;46:719–30.
47. Guinet F, Carniel E, Leclercq A. Transfusion-transmitted Yersinia enterocolitica sepsis. Clin Infect Dis 2011;53:583–91.
48. Kuehnert MJ, Roth VR, Haley NR, et al. Transfusion-transmitted bacterial infection in the United States, 1998 through 2000. Transfusion 2001;41:1493–9.
49. Kekre N, Tokessy M, Mallick R, et al. Is cytomegalovirus testing of blood products still needed for hematopoietic stem cell transplant recipients in the era of universal leukoreduction? Biol Blood Marrow Transplant 2013;19:1719–24.

50. Herwaldt BL, Linden JV, Bosserman E, et al. Transfusion-associated babesiosis in the United States: a description of cases. Ann Intern Med 2011;155:509–19.

51. Fatalities reported to FDA following blood collection and transfusion. Available at: http://www.fda.gov/downloads/BiologicsBloodVaccines/SafetyAvailability/ReportaProblem/TransfusionDonationFatalities/UCM459461.pdf. Accessed September 2, 2015.

52. Alter HJ, Klein HG. The hazards of blood transfusion in historical perspective. Blood 2008;112:2617–26.

53. Zou S, Stramer SL, Dodd RY. Donor testing and risk: current prevalence, incidence, and residual risk of transfusion-transmissible agents in US allogeneic donations. Transfus Med Rev 2012;26:119–28.

54. Montgomery SP, Brown JA, Kuehnert M, et al. Transfusion-associated transmission of West Nile virus, United States 2003 through 2005. Transfusion 2006;46:2038–46.

55. Biggerstaff BJ, Petersen LR. Estimated risk of transmission of the West Nile virus through blood transfusion in the US, 2002. Transfusion 2003;43:1007–17.

56. Dodd RY, Foster GA, Stramer SL. Keeping blood transfusion safe from West Nile virus: American Red Cross experience, 2003 to 2012. Transfus Med Rev 2015;29:153–61.

57. Levi JE, Nishiya A, Felix AC, et al. Real-time symptomatic case of transfusion-transmitted dengue. Transfusion 2015;55:961–4.

58. Petersen LR, Epstein JS. Chikungunya virus: new risk to transfusion safety in the Americas. Transfusion 2014;54:1911–5.

59. Arellanos-Soto D, B-d l Cruz V, Mendoza-Tavera N, et al. Constant risk of dengue virus infection by blood transfusion in an endemic area in Mexico. Transfus Med 2015;25:122–4.

60. Chiu CY, Bres V, Yu G, et al. Genomic assays for identification of chikungunya virus in blood donors, Puerto Rico, 2014. Emerg Infect Dis 2015;21:1409–13.

61. Keil SD, Bengrine A, Bowen R, et al. Inactivation of viruses in platelet and plasma products using a riboflavin-and-UV-based photochemical treatment. Transfusion 2015;55:1736–44.

62. Knutson F, Osselaer J, Pierelli L, et al. A prospective, active haemovigilance study with combined cohort analysis of 19 175 transfusions of platelet components prepared with amotosalen-UVA photochemical treatment. Vox Sang 2015;109(4):343–52.

63. Toy P, Gajic O, Bacchetti P, et al. Transfusion-related acute lung injury: incidence and risk factors. Blood 2012;119:1757–67.

64. Goldman M, Webert KE, Arnold DM, et al. Proceedings of a consensus conference: towards an understanding of TRALI. Transfus Med Rev 2005;19:2–31.

65. Vlaar AP, Juffermans NP. Transfusion-related acute lung injury: a clinical review. Lancet 2013;382:984–94.

66. Peters AL, van Hezel ME, Juffermans NP, et al. Pathogenesis of non-antibody mediated transfusion-related acute lung injury from bench to bedside. Blood Rev 2015;29:51–61.

67. Endres RO, Kleinman SH, Carrick DM, et al. Identification of specificities of antibodies against human leukocyte antigens in blood donors. Transfusion 2010;50:1749–60.

68. Wiersum-Osselton JC, Middelburg RA, Beckers EA, et al. Male-only fresh-frozen plasma for transfusion-related acute lung injury prevention: before-and-after comparative cohort study. Transfusion 2011;51:1278–83.

69. Khan SY, Kelher MR, Heal JM, et al. Soluble CD40 ligand accumulates in stored blood components, primes neutrophils through CD40, and is a potential cofactor in the development of transfusion-related acute lung injury. Blood 2006;108: 2455–62.

70. Silliman CC, Fung YL, Ball JB, et al. Transfusion-related acute lung injury (TRALI): current concepts and misconceptions. Blood Rev 2009;23:245–55.

71. Raval JS, Mazepa MA, Russell SL, et al. Passive reporting greatly underestimates the rate of transfusion-associated circulatory overload after platelet transfusion. Vox Sang 2015;108:387–92.

72. Narick C, Triulzi DJ, Yazer MH. Transfusion-associated circulatory overload after plasma transfusion. Transfusion 2012;52:160–5.

73. Tobian AA, Sokoll LJ, Tisch DJ, et al. N-terminal pro-brain natriuretic peptide is a useful diagnostic marker for transfusion-associated circulatory overload. Transfusion 2008;48:1143–50.

74. Zhou L, Giacherio D, Cooling L, et al. Use of B-natriuretic peptide as a diagnostic marker in the differential diagnosis of transfusion-associated circulatory overload. Transfusion 2005;45:1056–63.

75. Li G, Daniels CE, Kojicic M, et al. The accuracy of natriuretic peptides (brain natriuretic peptide and N-terminal pro-brain natriuretic) in the differentiation between transfusion-related acute lung injury and transfusion-related circulatory overload in the critically ill. Transfusion 2009;49:13–20.

76. Ohto H, Anderson KC. Survey of transfusion-associated graft-versus-host disease in immunocompetent recipients. Transfus Med Rev 1996;10:31–43.

77. Uchida S, Tadokoro K, Takahashi M, et al. Analysis of 66 patients definitive with transfusion-associated graft-versus-host disease and the effect of universal irradiation of blood. Transfus Med 2013;23:416–22.

78. Kopolovic I, Ostro J, Tsubota H, et al. A systematic review of transfusion-associated graft-versus-host disease. Blood 2015;126:406–14.

79. Akahoshi M, Takanashi M, Masuda M, et al. A case of transfusion-associated graft-versus-host disease not prevented by white cell-reduction filters. Transfusion 1992;32:169–72.

80. Hayashi H, Nishiuchi T, Tamura H, et al. Transfusion-associated graft-versus-host disease caused by leukocyte-filtered stored blood. Anesthesiology 1993;79: 1419–21.

81. Metcalfe P. Platelet antigens and antibody detection. Vox Sang 2004;87(Suppl 1): 82–6.

82. Waters AH. Post-transfusion purpura. Blood Rev 1989;3:83–7.

83. Lubenow N, Eichler P, Albrecht D, et al. Very low platelet counts in post-transfusion purpura falsely diagnosed as heparin-induced thrombocytopenia. Report of four cases and review of literature. Thromb Res 2000;100:115–25.

84. Weisberg LJ, Linker CA. Prednisone therapy of post-transfusion purpura. Ann Intern Med 1984;100:76–7.

85. Hamblin TJ, Naorose Abidi SM, Nee PA, et al. Successful treatment of post-transfusion purpura with high dose immunoglobulins after lack of response to plasma exchange. Vox Sang 1985;49:164–7.

86. Mueller-Eckhardt C, Kuenzlen E, Thilo-Korner D, et al. High-dose intravenous immunoglobulin for post-transfusion purpura. N Engl J Med 1983;308:287.

87. Mirski MA, Lele AV, Fitzsimmons L, et al. Diagnosis and treatment of vascular air embolism. Anesthesiology 2007;106:164–77.

Red Blood Cell Antibodies in Hematology/Oncology Patients

Interpretation of Immunohematologic Tests and Clinical Significance of Detected Antibodies

Jeanne E. Hendrickson, MD[a,b,]*, Christopher A. Tormey, MD[a,c]

KEYWORDS

- Red blood cell autoantibodies • Red blood cell alloantibodies • Alloimmunization
- Immunohematology • Compatibility testing • Blood banking
- Hematology/oncology disorders

KEY POINTS

- Many immunohematologic tests performed by blood banks, including antibody screening, direct antiglobulin tests, eluates, and minor antigen phenotyping, are relevant to hematology/oncology patients.
- Cold and warm autoantibodies may mediate intravascular or extravascular autoimmune hemolysis in hematology/oncology patients.
- Transfused individuals with hematologic/oncologic disorders may develop red blood cell alloantibodies, which can complicate pretransfusion testing, delay blood product availability, and lead to transfusion reactions.
- Several strategies exist to prevent the development of blood group alloantibodies in transfused hematology/oncology groups.

INTRODUCTION

Among the aspects of care rendered to patients with hematologic/oncologic disorders, blood transfusion is common. However, the tests that form the basis for transfusion compatibility and antibody identification are not always well understood, nor are their interpretations always straightforward. This article:

Conflicts of Interest: The authors have no conflicts to disclose relevant to this article.
[a] Department of Laboratory Medicine, Yale University School of Medicine, 333 Cedar Street, New Haven, CT 06520, USA; [b] Department of Pediatrics, Yale University School of Medicine, 333 Cedar Street, New Haven, CT 06520, USA; [c] Pathology and Laboratory Medicine Service, VA Connecticut Healthcare System, 950 Campbell Avenue, West Haven, CT 06516, USA
* Corresponding author. Department of Laboratory Medicine, 333 Cedar Street, PO Box 208035, New Haven, CT 06520.
E-mail address: jeanne.hendrickson@yale.edu

Hematol Oncol Clin N Am 30 (2016) 635–651
http://dx.doi.org/10.1016/j.hoc.2016.01.006
0889-8588/16/$ – see front matter © 2016 Elsevier Inc. All rights reserved.

hemonc.theclinics.com

1. Reviews immunohematologic tests performed by transfusion services
2. Describes how autoimmune hemolytic anemias (AIHA) are characterized by auto-antibodies detected
3. Outlines red blood cell (RBC) alloimmunization rates described in various hemato-logic/oncologic patient populations and the potential ramifications of these alloantibodies
4. Presents potential strategies to mitigate RBC alloimmunization

BASIC TESTS OF COMPATIBILITY IN THE BLOOD BANK

For hematology/oncology patients, one of the most commonly performed tests is the type and screen. In this testing, an individual's ABO and Rh(D) status is determined (the type) and the presence/absence of autoantibodies or alloantibodies is established (the screen).

Principle of Hemagglutination and Testing Platforms in the Blood Bank

Of the tests to be discussed later, a basic tenet inherent to all is mixing patient spec-imen (plasma or RBCs) with a reagent to examine for a reaction. Positive testing in the blood bank setting typically is reflected as hemagglutination. The strength of the agglutination reaction is graded on a 0 to 4+ scale, with 0 indicating a negative test (ie, no agglutination) and 4+ indicating an overwhelmingly positive reaction.

Hemagglutination can take place via several laboratory platforms. Historically, compatibility testing was performed in glass or plastic tubes, with patient specimen and reagent added, and, after several incubation and wash steps, observation for agglutination. Given the moderate sensitivity and laborious nature of the tube method, several technological advancements were subsequently introduced. Although still based on the fundamental principle of agglutination, platforms such as automated gel columns have been developed to further augment a blood bank's ability to detect RBC antibodies.[1-3] More recently, automated platforms involving solid phase RBC adherence (wherein a patient's plasma is mixed with immobilized RBC antigens on a plate or well) have been accepted into clinical practice.[4] Although gel and solid phase platforms have increased sensitivity compared with tube methods, this comes with a concomitant increase in false-positive reactions.

ABO and Rh(D) Blood Group Phenotyping

The ABO system, representing a series of carbohydrate antigens on the RBC surface, is the single most important blood group family for transfusion compatibility. Infusion of ABO incompatible blood components can result in severe hemolytic reactions, morbidity, and death.[5] ABO antigens are particularly problematic because individuals lacking a given antigen within this system make a corresponding antibody from early in life without the need for prior RBC exposure via transfusion or pregnancy. As such, thorough and reliable mechanisms for determining an individual's ABO status are crit-ical for compatibility.

Blood banks typically perform 2 steps in determination of an individual's ABO sta-tus: forward grouping for the presence or absence of A or B antigens (informally referred to as the front type) and reverse grouping for the presence of anti-A or anti-B antibodies in plasma (informally referred to as the back type). The front type involves detection of A or B antigen using reagent antibodies directed against these targets. The back type is meant to serve as a confirmation of the results of the front type and is based on the previously described principle that an individual lacking a given ABO antigen should have a detectable antibody against that antigen.

In terms of clinical significance, the Rh blood group antigen system is the second most important after ABO. Unlike ABO antigens, which are carbohydrate in nature, Rh antigens are polypeptide and typically require a previous exposure before induction of an alloantibody. Also unlike the ABO system, the Rh system is highly complex with more than 30 unique antigens.[6] However, during routine practice, blood banks only test for the presence or absence of a single antigen in the Rh system: Rh(D).

Phenotyping for the other, non-Rh(D), minor blood group antigens may also be completed for select patient populations. Such phenotyping for antigens including C/c, E/e, and K is also typically done by mixing patient RBCs with antisera against these antigens and can be completed with tube or automated methods. As described in more detail later, determining an extended antigen phenotype is typically reserved for patients at high risk for RBC alloimmunization.

COMPLEX TESTS OF COMPATIBILITY AND/OR ANTIBODY IDENTIFICATION IN THE BLOOD BANK

Besides the basic tests of compatibility described earlier, blood banks are often called on to perform more additional tests to identify autoantibodies and alloantibodies (described later and in **Table 1**).

Indirect Antiglobulin Test

The type and screen is the most frequently performed test in the blood bank. When providers order a screen, blood banks are performing an indirect antiglobulin test (IAT) to identify possible autoantibodies or alloantibodies in patients' plasma. **Fig. 1** provides an overview of the IAT, which involves mixture of patient plasma with screening cells expressing various combinations of clinically relevant, non-ABO antigens. IATs are designed primarily to detect immunoglobulin (Ig) G class antibodies.[7] If an IAT is negative, then there is no evidence for an existing autoantibody or alloantibody in the patient's plasma and blood banks will provide RBCs for transfusion. However, if an IAT is positive, blood banks must identify the cause of that positive reaction such that compatible units for RBC transfusion can be provided. As such, blood banks reflex positive IATs to RBC antibody panel testing.

Identification of Red Blood Cell Antibodies by Panel Testing

The panel assay is performed using a mixture of patient plasma and numerous reagent cell lines. In many ways, panel testing is analogous to the simple IAT screen, with the most significant difference being the number of reagent cells used (10–12 in the panel vs 2–4 in the screen). Selection of a larger number of reagent cells in the panel helps blood banks more clearly identify the antibodies driving the positive reaction.

Note that not every positive IAT reaction is attributable to an alloantibody. Warm-reactive autoantibodies frequently give rise to positive screening tests.[8] However, compared with the results seen with an alloantibody, panels for patients with autoantibodies generally show panagglutination; that is, reactivity with every reagent cell tested. Such a finding typically warrants the performance of a direct antiglobulin test (DAT).

Direct Antiglobulin Test

The DAT is a highly sensitive assay used to detect antibody or complement bound to the RBC surface. As shown in **Fig. 2**, DATs are typically 2-step tests, with the first step involving a polyspecific reagent detecting either IgG or complement component C3 on

Table 1
The expected results of immunohematologic tests in various autoimmune and alloimmune settings

	IAT[a]	RBC Panel	Antibody Identified in RBC Panel	DAT[a] IgG | C3	RBC Elution	Antibody Identified in RBC Elution	Cold Screen	DL Test
Alloimmune Processes								
Primary immune response to pregnancy or transfusion	+	+	Specific IgG alloantibody	−/− | −/−	−	None	−	−
Anamnestic response or delayed hemolytic transfusion reaction	+	+	Specific IgG alloantibody	−/+ | −/+	+	Specific IgG alloantibody	−	−
Autoimmune Processes								
Warm autoimmune hemolytic anemia	+/−	+/−	Panagglutinin	+ | −/+	+	Panagglutinin	−	−
Cold agglutinin disease	−	−	None	− | +	−	None	+	−
Mixed autoimmune hemolytic anemia	+	+	Panagglutinin	+ | +	+	Panagglutinin	+	−
Paroxysmal cold hemoglobinuria	−	−	None	− | +	−	None	−	+

Abbreviations: DAT, direct antiglobulin test; DL, Donath-Landsteiner; IAT, indirect antiglobulin test; IgG, immunoglobulin G.

[a] For results indicating '+/−' or '−/+', testing in this setting could give rise to either negative or positive results, depending on the clinical scenario and the antibodies involved. For DATs, expected results of IgG testing are the top line result, whereas C3 results are on the bottom line.

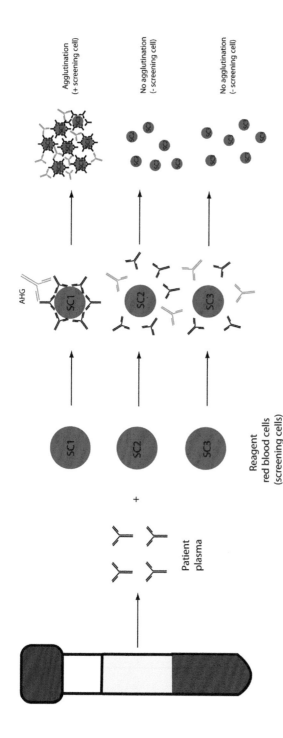

Fig. 1. The IAT. This assay is used primarily for the detection of IgG class autoantibodies and/or alloantibodies in patient plasma. It involves a mixture of a patient's plasma with reagent screening cells (SCs) expressing a variety of blood group antigens, followed by the addition of anti–human globulin (AHG). A positive IAT manifests as an agglutination reaction.

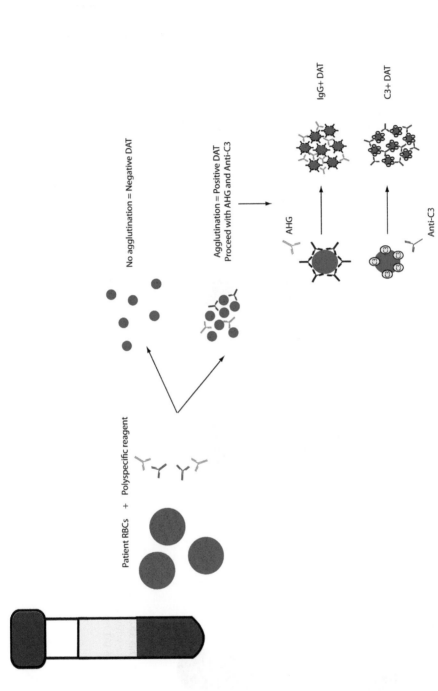

Fig. 2. The DAT. This assay is used primarily for the determination of whether IgG or complement component C3 is bound to a patient's RBCs; the primary end point is agglutination. The DAT is a 2-part test with the first step involving a mixture of patient's specimen with a polyspecific reagent capable of agglutinating either IgG and/or C3-coated RBCs. If the polyspecific step shows RBC agglutination, then specific testing using AHG or anti-C3 must be used to determine whether IgG, C3, or both are coating the patient's RBCs.

the RBC surface. Agglutination with polyspecific reagents requires additional testing to determine whether IgG, C3, or both are on the RBC surface.

A positive DAT with IgG or C3 may be suggestive of a hemolytic picture, with IgG reactivity often correlating with a warm-reactive antibody/extravascular hemolysis and C3 reactivity typically correlating with a cold-reactive antibody/intravascular hemolysis. However, as a highly sensitive test, the DAT can also be prone to false-positive reactions. Causes of false-positive DATs (ie, agglutination in the absence of immune-mediated hemolysis) include the following:

- Administration of drugs that modify the RBC surface (eg, antibiotics)
- Polyclonal hypergammaglobulinemia
- Previous transfusions
- Severe RBC rouleaux

Red Blood Cell Elution

RBC elution is used to evaluate the specificity of an antibody bound to the RBC surface. Although several laboratory techniques are available to help liberate antibodies from RBCs, many blood banks use an acid elution approach for optimal removal. As outlined in **Fig. 3**, the interaction between RBC and antibody is weakened in an acidic environment, allowing formerly bound RBC antibodies to accumulate in the plasma. Specimens are then centrifuged and the supernatant plasma removed. The antibody-concentrated supernatant is then reacted with an RBC panel to identify the antibody specificity.

In the setting of AIHA, in which autoantibodies are targeting highly conserved portions of the RBC membrane,[9] RBC elution studies show panagglutination. In contrast, in the setting of alloimmune hemolysis (eg, following an incompatible RBC transfusion), RBC elution studies typically show reactivity for a specific non-ABO antigen. Note that elution studies are most useful for IgG-positive DATs. C3-positive DATs are frequently associated with IgM antibodies; such antibodies are poorly eluted from the RBC surface and, in most blood bank settings, few reagents exist to detect bound IgM.

Cold Autoantibody Screen, Thermal Amplitude, and Titers

Cold autoantibodies are classically IgM and may be difficult to detect by standard blood bank testing. Therefore, cold screens have been developed to help identify the presence/absence of a cold autoantibody as well as possible targets of the autoantibodies on the RBC surface. In a cold autoantibody screen, a patient's plasma specimen (collected and maintained at 37°C) is subsequently mixed with adult screening cells (harboring the I antigen), cord-blood RBCs (harboring the i antigen), and the patient's RBCs (to determine whether any reactivity against self is demonstrable); all testing is done at 4°C. In most forms of cold agglutinin disease (CAD) in adults, cold autoantibodies should show strong reactivity against self and RBCs possessing the I antigen. Such reactivity classically has been described in CAD associated with *Mycoplasma pneumoniae* infections. In contrast, cold autoantibodies showing strong reactivity against self and i-positive RBCs may suggest CAD associated with Epstein-Barr virus infection.[10]

When clinical suspicion exists for CAD, the cold screen is only the first step because many patients can possess clinically insignificant cold autoantibodies. Differentiating a significant from insignificant cold agglutinin requires clinical correlation in addition to examining the thermal amplitude of the autoantibody and its titer. Thermal amplitude studies involve incubating the patient's plasma with screening cells at temperatures

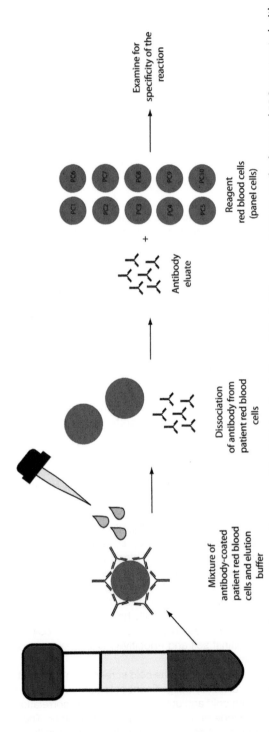

Fig. 3. RBC elution studies are used to evaluate a positive DAT showing IgG reactivity. In this assay, a patient's antibody-coated RBCs are treated with a buffer that causes dissociation of the antibodies from the RBC surface. This concentrated RBC eluate is then reacted against reagent panel cells to determine the specificity of the autoantibodies or alloantibodies.

ranging from 0°C to 4°C through 35°C to 37°C. Most clinically significant cold autoantibodies show reactivity (ie, hemagglutination) at temperatures greater than 27°C to 30°C. Regarding titers, several dilutions of patient plasma are mixed with screening cells at 4°C to determine the strength of the autoantibody. Although no formal guidelines exist, reports in the literature suggest that titers of greater than 1:64 to 1:256 are consistent with clinically significant CAD.[9]

Donath-Landsteiner Test

Paroxysmal cold hemoglobinuria (PCH) is a rare cold AIHA. Most often encountered after infection or vaccination in children, and presenting with severe intravascular hemolysis, PCH is caused by an IgG autoantibody (referred to as biphasic hemolysin) targeting the high-incidence P antigen.[11] The DAT is typically positive for complement only, because the cold-reactive IgG autoantibody dissociates from the patient's RBCs at the warmer temperature at which the DAT is performed. Physiologically, the biphasic nature of PCH is manifested by autoantibodies binding to RBCs at cold temperatures and fixing complement (phase I). Then, as RBCs warm back toward 37°C, fixed complement is within its optimal thermal range and intravascular RBC hemolysis ensues (phase II).[12] The Donath-Landsteiner test thus involves incubating the patient's plasma with control RBCs at a very cold temperature (typically 0°C –4°C) allowing any cold-reactive IgG autoantibodies to bind and fix complement. This specimen is then incubated at 37°C, allowing fixed complement to lyse the RBCs. When a PCH autoantibody is present, there should be gross hemolysis observed in the plasma supernatant of specimens incubated at 0°C to 4°C followed by 37°C.

Summary for Complex Tests of Compatibility and/or Antibody Identification

The tests described earlier are used in the assessment of hematology/oncology patients who require transfusion care, or in whom an alloimmune or autoimmune process is suspected. A detailed description of the further diagnosis and treatment of AIHA is beyond the scope of this article and the reader is referred to the June 2015 edition of *Hematology/Oncology Clinics of North America* for in-depth reviews of warm and cold AIHA.[8,13] Because of these recent reviews of AIHA, the remainder of this article focuses on the alloimmune response to blood group antigens in patients with hematologic/oncologic disorders.

RED BLOOD CELL ALLOIMMUNIZATION IN HEMATOLOGY/ONCOLOGY DISORDERS AND ITS CLINICAL SIGNIFICANCE

Given the close relationship between transfusion therapy and the management of hematologic/oncologic disorders, there have been several studies examining rates of blood group alloantibody development in these diseases (described later and in **Table 2**). As a comparison, a study of nearly 20,000 transfused male veterans reported an alloantibody prevalence of 2.4%.[14]

Alloimmunization in Hematologic or Oncologic Disorders (Nonhemoglobinopathies)

Myelodysplastic syndromes, acute myeloid leukemia, and aplastic anemia

There have been several studies of RBC alloimmunization among patients with myelodysplastic syndromes (MDS) and/or myelodysplastic/myeloproliferative neoplasms. These investigations have shown that 15% to 59% of patients with MDS or MDS-related disorders can develop alloantibodies.[15,16] In comparison, patients with acute myeloid leukemia (AML) have been found to have alloimmunization rates ranging from 3% to 16%,[16,17] whereas those with aplastic anemia (AA) show rates of about 11% to

Table 2	
RBC alloimmunization rates reported in various hematologic and oncologic disorders	
Disease/Disorder	**Reported Alloimmunization Rates (%)**
Acute lymphoid leukemia	<1
Acute myeloid leukemia	3–16
Aplastic anemia	11–14
Hematopoietic progenitor cell transplant	1–4
Hodgkin lymphoma	<1
Non-Hodgkin lymphoma	2–3
Myelodysplastic syndromes[a]	15–59
Solid tumors	1–10
Sickle cell disease[a]	19–43
Thalassemia[a]	5–45

Rates indicated in the table represent historical reports from large studies.

[a] For the disorders with an asterisk, studies have shown that phenotypic or genotypic matching for non-ABO antigens may decrease alloimmunization rates, potentially to levels less than the values reported in the table.

14%.[16,18] Consequences of the alloimmunization rates in these patients include delays in the timely provision of compatible blood products and the potential for alloantibodies to complicate stem cell transplantation. Based on these hazards, some investigators have advocated prophylactic antigen matching for patients with myeloid disorders or AA. For instance, when such a strategy was used in the setting of MDS, alloantibody development rates decreased.[15]

Acute lymphocytic leukemia, Hodgkin lymphoma, and non-Hodgkin lymphoma
There have been few studies on alloimmunization rates in individuals with immature or mature lymphoid neoplasms and, overall, very low rates of alloimmunization have been observed, ranging from 0% of patients with acute lymphocytic leukemia (ALL) and Hodgkin lymphoma[16,18] to about 2% to 3% in patients with various non-Hodgkin lymphomas and plasma cell neoplasms.[16] A recent study found that lymphoproliferative disorders in general tend to be associated with the absence of alloimmunization.[19] It has been hypothesized that lower rates of alloimmunization in such disorders may be attributable to the chemotherapy regimens used for these entities, or impaired immune function associated with the disorders themselves.[18,19]

Bone marrow/hematopoietic progenitor cell transplant
Because transfusion support is a critical component of progenitor cell transplantation, several studies have examined the rates at which individuals develop alloantibodies in the posttransplant period. Rates of new antibody development (ie, antibodies attributable specifically to RBC transfusions posttransplant) are low, with a small percentage of recipients becoming alloimmunized.[20–22] At least 1 study indicated that recipients of ABO-mismatched allogeneic transplants may be at higher risk for developing blood group antibodies.[22]

Solid tumors and general patients with cancer
Despite patients with solid tumors frequently undergoing RBC transfusion, there have been few studies examining alloimmunization rates in such individuals. Two of the larger studies have produced disparate results, with alloimmunization rates ranging

from very low (<1% of transfused patients)[23] to moderately high (about 8%–10% of patients).[24] One large case-control study found that history of a solid malignancy was more likely to be associated with RBC alloimmunization.[19] However, a subsequent investigation of alloimmunized patients with nonhematologic malignancies failed to identify risk factors that might be associated with an alloantibody responder status among such individuals.[25]

Alloimmunization in Hemoglobinopathies

Sickle cell disease

Transfusions are increasingly being utilized in patients with sickle cell disease (SCD) to prevent and treat disease associated complications (See Chou ST, Fasano RM: Management of Patients with Sickle Cell Disease Using Transfusion Therapy: Guidelines and Complications, in this issue).[26,27] One significant transfusion-associated risk is RBC alloimmunization, with patients with SCD having rates of 19% to 43%.[28,29] Recent studies suggest potentially lower rates of alloimmunization (despite increased blood product exposure) in patients with SCD undergoing chronic RBC exchange transfusions compared with those receiving simple transfusions.[30,31] Antibodies most prevalent in patients with SCD are those against Rh, K, and Jk^b antigens reflecting, in part, the antigenic differences between blood donors and SCD recipients.[32] Alloimmunized patients with SCD often have coexistent RBC autoantibodies.

RBC alloantibodies may have far-reaching consequences in patients with SCD, including acute or delayed hemolytic reactions; bystander hemolysis; and, in women of childbearing age, hemolytic disease of the fetus and newborn (HDFN).[33,34] Delayed hemolytic transfusion reactions (DHTRs) and bystander hemolysis are particularly problematic in patients with SCD. Although the pathophysiology of bystander hemolysis is not fully understood, this complication may occur approximately 5 to 14 days after the transfusion of seemingly compatible RBCs. Destruction of the transfused RBCs, in addition to the patient's own RBCs, ensues with severe anemia and death potentially resulting. These reactions may initially present with pain or fever, and be misdiagnosed as simple vaso-occlusive crises. A recent study of 220 adults with SCD documented that up to 48% of DHTRs were not diagnosed at the time of the event.[35] Such reactions tend to occur in alloimmunized patients, although RBC alloantibodies are not detected in all reactions. Recommended treatments of DHTRs with bystander hemolysis include avoiding further transfusions if possible (in the acute phase of such reactions) and considering treatment with steroids and/or intravenous immunoglobulin; treatment with an erythropoiesis-stimulating agent and iron may also be useful.[36] Emerging data suggest that pretreatment with rituximab may prevent or mitigate such reactions in a subset of patients who have previously had bystander hemolysis.[37] However, controlled trials are lacking in this area. In addition, RBC alloantibodies may also delay or prevent potentially lifesaving transfusions. A recent study correlated RBC alloimmunization with overall worse survival in patients with SCD.[38]

A subset of patients with SCD never become alloimmunized despite exposure to hundreds of RBC units; this observation has resulted in a search to identify immunologic or genetic signatures of responder and nonresponder patients.[39] In addition to genetic or immunologic markers, the inflammatory status of a recipient at the time of RBC exposure may determine whether an alloantibody is formed to that particular transfusion. Two recent publications implicate inflammation in patients with SCD as contributing to RBC alloimmunization.[38,40] Past studies in animals[41] as well as in patients without SCD[42] have also implicated inflammation at the time of transfusion as a risk factor for RBC alloimmunization.

Thalassemia

Chronic RBC transfusions are essential for patients with some forms of β-thalassemia. Unlike patients with SCD, patients with thalassemia often begin transfusion therapy early in life. Although hemosiderosis and infectious disease transmission have historically been among the leading transfusion-associated concerns for patients with thalassemia, RBC alloimmunization is increasingly being recognized as a significant transfusion hazard. Reported rates of alloimmunization in patients with thalassemia major range from 5% to 45%.[43]

The worldwide distribution of patients with thalassemia major is broad, and alloimmunization rates vary by country because of the homogeneity of the donor/recipient population; the resources available in a particular country for antibody detection; and varying blood collection, processing, and matching techniques/protocols. The US Centers for Disease Control and Prevention Thalassemia Blood Safety Network recently reported an alloimmunization rate of 21% in North American patients, with commonly detected antibodies including anti-C, anti-E, and anti-K.[44] Studies originating in Europe have reported alloimmunization rates of about 5% to 25%,[45,46] whereas in the Middle East and India rates of 4% to 30% have been observed.[47,48] In these European, Middle Eastern, and Indian studies, the most common antibodies detected were directed against K and Rh antigens. Chinese patients with thalassemia are also likely to have antibodies directed against antigens in the Miltenberger family.[43]

A few factors, including age at initial RBC exposure and the presence or absence of a spleen, have been studied with regard to alloimmunization in patients with thalassemia. Younger age at the time of initial RBC exposure correlates (in some studies) with a lower likelihood of alloimmunization.[44,46,49] These findings are not unique to patients with thalassemia, with similar trends reported in patients with SCD.[50] The immunologic mechanisms behind these observations are not fully understood, although tolerance to RBC antigens has been reported to occur in a murine model of RBC alloimmunization.[51] Another factor that has received much attention in recent years involves whether the presence of a spleen affects RBC alloimmunization in patients with thalassemia. Conflicting reports exist,[48,49,52–54] with variables to consider in interpreting the existing data including the indication for splenectomy (usually high transfusion requirements) and the transfusion burden, which has also been found to correlate with alloimmunization risk. Further, the timing of the splenectomy in relationship to initial RBC exposure is also presumably important.

Another consideration in transfusion of patients with thalassemia is blood product modification. Most blood transfused in the United States is prestorage filter leukoreduced. Although the impact of leukoreduction on RBC alloimmunization is not clear, all US sites within the Thalassemia Clinical Research Network report using leukoreduced blood.[44] One site also reported transfusing washed RBCs, a process that damages RBCs and should be reserved for the rare recipients with significant allergies to proteins in the plasma of an RBC unit. Washing, via RBC damage, could theoretically alter risks for RBC alloimmunization.

RED BLOOD CELL ALLOANTIBODY MITIGATION STRATEGIES

Avoiding RBC transfusion altogether is one strategy to minimize RBC alloimmunization, although this is not often feasible in hematology/oncology patients. Thus, the main strategy used to minimize RBC alloimmunization is the transfusion of RBCs that are at least partially matched between donor and recipient. However, beyond ABO and Rh(D), there is much variation in the degree of matching that occurs between blood donors and recipients.

Phenotypic matching for C/c, E/e, and K for patients with SCD was first suggested in the 1990s as a strategy to decrease alloimmunization rates; these antigens were selected given their immunogenicity as well as differences in expression between blood donors and SCD recipients.[32] In 2014, the National Institutes of Health SCD Management guidelines[55] formally recommended that patients with SCD receive RBCs prophylactically matched at C/c, E/e, and K/k.[56] Several studies have shown that providing partially phenotypically matched RBCs to patients with SCD decreases RBC alloimmunization,[57–59] although other studies have shown high rates of alloimmunization despite prophylactic phenotypic matching.[60,61] This persistence of high alloimmunization rates despite phenotypic matching is caused, at least in part, by the presence of Rh variants in patients with SCD and/or blood donors.

Given the limitations associated with serologic antigen phenotyping, genotyping (ie, the use of DNA-based techniques to evaluate the expression of blood group antigens) has become more widely applied to transfusion medicine.[62] Several studies have investigated the logistical considerations of genotyping patients with SCD and their blood donors, with the goal of decreasing inadvertent exposure to foreign RBC antigens. Improved transfusion outcomes have been reported in some studies in which genotype is used to predict phenotype.[63] However, the provision of RBCs genetically matched at all antigenic sites remains impossible, because matching at one site may increase the likelihood of mismatching at another site.

Although no US guidelines exist, the selection of RBCs matched beyond Rh(D) may decrease rates of RBC alloimmunization in thalassemic populations. Phenotypically matched RBCs were reported to be associated with a low rate of alloimmunization (2.8%) in one thalassemia study, compared with a rate of 33% before the use of phenotypically matched, leukoreduced RBCs.[64] A larger study showed a 3.7% rate of RBC alloimmunization in thalassemia recipients of RBCs matched at ABO, Rh, and K, compared with a 22.6% rate in recipients receiving only ABO-matched and Rh(D)-matched RBCs.[46] Further, another study reported lower RBC alloimmunization rates (8.3%) in patients with thalassemia receiving blood from a limited number of donors, compared with those not in a limited donor program (21.6%).[65] Alloimmunized hematology/oncology patients without SCD or thalassemia who are at increased risk of forming additional alloantibodies with blood exposure may also benefit from receiving RBCs matched beyond ABO and Rh(D). Further, some centers provide phenotypically matched RBCs for patients with AIHA to minimize the formation of RBC alloantibodies; such alloantibodies may be difficult to detect in the presence of AIHA.[66]

Other strategies for mitigating the dangers of RBC alloantibodies include increasing awareness about the importance of an accurate transfusion history. Antibodies may evanesce, or decrease to below the level of detection by a hospital transfusion service[67]; as an example, only 18 patients with SCD had detectable RBC alloantibodies on enrollment in the PROACTIVE (Preventing Acute Chest Syndrome by Transfusion) study, but 34 patients had an antibody history.[68] Once detected, a clinically significant RBC alloantibody must always be honored (ie, RBCs lacking the cognate antigen should be selected for transfusion), regardless of whether the antibody is currently detected. However, at present there are no US-wide blood bank databases from which to retrieve historical RBC alloantibody information. Centralized blood bank databases and/or Web-based antibody registries could significantly increase transfusion safety.

SUMMARY

Although transfusions are essential to the treatment of many hematology/oncology diseases, they are not risk free. Alloimmunization is a significant risk of transfusions, and is the second leading cause of transfusion-associated death in the United States.[69] A better understanding of testing completed in the blood bank will allow hematology/oncology providers to make informed decisions on the risk/benefit ratio of transfusion for their individual patients. Further, this understanding will allow improved communication between hematology/oncology providers and the transfusion service (and vice versa) in instances of transfusion histories, new antibody formation, and unexpected adverse transfusion sequelae. Joint advocacy for RBC alloantibody prevention and mitigation, on the parts of the hematology/oncology/transplant and the transfusion medicine communities alike, should be strived for as a patient safety initiative.

REFERENCES

1. Brumit MC, Stubbs JR. Conventional tube agglutination with polyethylene glycol versus Red Cell Affinity Column Technology (ReACT): a comparison of antibody detection methods. Ann Clin Lab Sci 2002;32(2):155–8.
2. Plapp FV, Rachel JM. Automation in blood banking. Machines for clumping, sticking, and gelling. Am J Clin Pathol 1992;98(4 Suppl 1):S17–21.
3. Morelati F, Revelli N, Maffei LM, et al. Evaluation of a new automated instrument for pretransfusion testing. Transfusion 1998;38(10):959–65.
4. Sallander S, Shanwell A, Aqvist M. Evaluation of a solid-phase test for erythrocyte antibody screening of pregnant women, patients and blood donors. Vox Sang 1996;71(4):221–5.
5. Simmons DP, Savage WJ. Hemolysis from ABO incompatibility. Hematol Oncol Clin North Am 2015;29(3):429–43.
6. Flegel WA. Molecular genetics and clinical applications for RH. Transfus Apheresis Sci 2011;44(1):81–91.
7. Downes KA, Shulman IA. Pretransfusion testing. In: Fung MK, editor. Technical manual. 18th edition. Bethesda (MD): AABB Press; 2014. p. 367–87.
8. Naik R. Warm autoimmune hemolytic anemia. Hematol Oncol Clin North Am 2015; 29(3):445–53.
9. Janvier D, Lam Y, Lopez I, et al. A major target for warm immunoglobulin G autoantibodies: the third external loop of Band 3. Transfusion 2013;53(9):1948–55.
10. Petz LD. Cold antibody autoimmune hemolytic anemias. Blood Rev 2008;22(1): 1–15.
11. Shanbhag S, Spivak J. Paroxysmal cold hemoglobinuria. Hematol Oncol Clin North Am 2015;29(3):473–8.
12. Sanford KW, Roseff SD. Detection and significance of Donath-Landsteiner antibodies in a 5-year-old female presenting with hemolytic anemia. Lab Med 2010;41:209–12.
13. Berentsen S, Randen U, Tjonnfjord GE. Cold agglutinin-mediated autoimmune hemolytic anemia. Hematol Oncol Clin North Am 2015;29(3):455–71.
14. Tormey CA, Fisk J, Stack G. Red blood cell alloantibody frequency, specificity, and properties in a population of male military veterans. Transfusion 2008; 48(10):2069–76.
15. Guelsin GA, Rodrigues C, Visentainer JE, et al. Molecular matching for Rh and K reduces red blood cell alloimmunisation in patients with myelodysplastic syndrome. Blood Transfus 2015;13(1):53–8.
16. Seyfried H, Walewska I. Analysis of immune response to red blood cell antigens in multitransfused patients with different diseases. Mater Med Pol 1990;22(1): 21–5.

17. Blumberg N, Heal JM, Gettings KF. WBC reduction of RBC transfusions is associated with a decreased incidence of RBC alloimmunization. Transfusion 2003; 43(7):945–52.

18. Blumberg N, Peck K, Ross K, et al. Immune response to chronic red blood cell transfusion. Vox Sang 1983;44(4):212–7.

19. Bauer MP, Wiersum-Osselton J, Schipperus M, et al. Clinical predictors of alloimmunization after red blood cell transfusion. Transfusion 2007;47(11):2066–71.

20. Perseghin P, Balduzzi A, Galimberti S, et al. Red blood cell support and alloimmunization rate against erythrocyte antigens in patients undergoing hematopoietic stem cell transplantation. Bone Marrow Transplant 2003;32(2):231–6.

21. Booth GS, Gehrie EA, Savani BN. Minor RBC Ab and allo-SCT. Bone Marrow Transplant 2014;49(3):456–7.

22. de la Rubia J, Arriaga F, Andreu R, et al. Development of non-ABO RBC alloantibodies in patients undergoing allogeneic HPC transplantation. Is ABO incompatibility a predisposing factor? Transfusion 2001;41(1):106–10.

23. Havemann H, Lichtiger B. Identification of previous erythrocyte alloimmunization and the type and screen at a large cancer center. A 4-year retrospective review. Cancer 1992;69(1):252–5.

24. Baby M, Fongoro S, Cisse M, et al. Frequency of red blood cell alloimmunization in polytransfused patients at the university teaching hospital of VMali. Transfus Clin Biol 2010;17(4):218–22 [in French].

25. Dinardo CL, Ito GM, Sampaio LR, et al. Study of possible clinical and laboratory predictors of alloimmunization against red blood cell antigens in cancer patients. Rev Bras Hematol Hemoter 2013;35(6):414–6.

26. DeBaun MR, Gordon M, McKinstry RC, et al. Controlled trial of transfusions for silent cerebral infarcts in sickle cell anemia. N Engl J Med 2014;371(8):699–710.

27. Beverung LM, Strouse JJ, Hulbert ML, et al. Health-related quality of life in children with sickle cell anemia: impact of blood transfusion therapy. Am J Hematol 2015;90(2):139–43.

28. Josephson CD, Su LL, Hillyer KL, et al. Transfusion in the patient with sickle cell disease: a critical review of the literature and transfusion guidelines. Transfus Med Rev 2007;21(2):118–33.

29. Aygun B, Padmanabhan S, Paley C, et al. Clinical significance of RBC alloantibodies and autoantibodies in sickle cell patients who received transfusions. Transfusion 2002;42(1):37–43.

30. Wahl SK, Garcia A, Hagar W, et al. Lower alloimmunization rates in pediatric sickle cell patients on chronic erythrocytapheresis compared to chronic simple transfusions. Transfusion 2012;52(12):2671–6.

31. Michot JM, Driss F, Guitton C, et al. Immunohematologic tolerance of chronic transfusion exchanges with erythrocytapheresis in sickle cell disease. Transfusion 2015;55(2):357–63.

32. Vichinsky EP, Earles A, Johnson RA, et al. Alloimmunization in sickle-cell-anemia and transfusion of racially unmatched blood. N Engl J Med 1990;322(23):1617–21.

33. King KE, Shirey RS, Lankiewicz MW, et al. Delayed hemolytic transfusion reactions in sickle cell disease: simultaneous destruction of recipients' red cells. Transfusion 1997;37(4):376–81.

34. Win N. Hyperhemolysis syndrome in sickle cell disease. Expert Rev Hematol 2009;2(2):111–5.

35. Vidler JB, Gardner K, Amenyah K, et al. Delayed haemolytic transfusion reaction in adults with sickle cell disease: a 5-year experience. Br J Haematol 2015; 169(5):746–53.

36. Gardner K, Hoppe C, Mijovic A, et al. How we treat delayed haemolytic transfusion reactions in patients with sickle cell disease. Br J Haematol 2015;170(6): 745–56.

37. Noizat-Pirenne F, Habibi A, Mekontso-Dessap A, et al. The use of rituximab to prevent severe delayed haemolytic transfusion reaction in immunized patients with sickle cell disease. Vox Sang 2015;108(3):262–7.

38. Telen MJ, Afenyi-Annan A, Garrett ME, et al. Alloimmunization in sickle cell disease: changing antibody specificities and association with chronic pain and decreased survival. Transfusion 2015;55(6 Pt 2):1378–87.

39. Kacker S, Ness PM, Savage WJ, et al. Economic evaluation of a hypothetical screening assay for alloimmunization risk among transfused patients with sickle cell disease. Transfusion 2014;54(8):2034–44.

40. Seferi I, Xhetani M, Face M, et al. Frequency and specificity of red cell antibodies in thalassemia patients in Albania. Int J Lab Hematol 2015;37(4):569–74.

41. Hendrickson JE, Desmarets M, Deshpande SS, et al. Recipient inflammation affects the frequency and magnitude of immunization to transfused red blood cells. Transfusion 2006;46(9):1526–36.

42. Papay P, Hackner K, Vogelsang H, et al. High risk of transfusion-induced alloimmunization of patients with inflammatory bowel disease. Am J Med 2012;125(7): 717.e1–8.

43. Matteocci A, Pierelli L. Red blood cell alloimmunization in sickle cell disease and in thalassaemia: current status, future perspectives and potential role of molecular typing. Vox Sang 2014;106(3):197–208.

44. Vichinsky E, Neumayr L, Trimble S, et al. Transfusion complications in thalassemia patients: a report from the Centers for Disease Control and Prevention (CME). Transfusion 2014;54(4):972–81 [quiz: 971].

45. Sirchia G, Zanella A, Parravicini A, et al. Red cell alloantibodies in thalassemia major. Results of an Italian cooperative study. Transfusion 1985;25(2):110–2.

46. Spanos T, Karageorga M, Ladis V, et al. Red cell alloantibodies in patients with thalassemia. Vox Sang 1990;58(1):50–5.

47. Ameen R, Al-Shemmari S, Al-Humood S, et al. RBC alloimmunization and autoimmunization among transfusion-dependent Arab thalassemia patients. Transfusion 2003;43(11):1604–10.

48. Azarkeivan A, Ansari S, Ahmadi MH, et al. Blood transfusion and alloimmunization in patients with thalassemia: multicenter study. Pediatr Hematol Oncol 2011;28(6):479–85.

49. Gupta R, Singh DK, Singh B, et al. Alloimmunization to red cells in thalassemics: emerging problem and future strategies. Transfus Apheresis Sci 2011;45(2): 167–70.

50. Tatari-Calderone Z, Minniti CP, Kratovil T, et al. rs660 polymorphism in Ro52 (SSA1; TRIM21) is a marker for age-dependent tolerance induction and efficiency of alloimmunization in sickle cell disease. Mol Immunol 2009;47(1):64–70.

51. Smith NH, Hod EA, Spitalnik SL, et al. Transfusion in the absence of inflammation induces antigen-specific tolerance to murine RBCs. Blood 2012;119(6):1566–9.

52. Thompson AA, Cunningham MJ, Singer ST, et al. Red cell alloimmunization in a diverse population of transfused patients with thalassaemia. Br J Haematol 2011;153(1):121–8.

53. Pahuja S, Pujani M, Gupta SK, et al. Alloimmunization and red cell autoimmuniza-tion in multitransfused thalassemics of Indian origin. Hematology 2010;15(3): 174–7.

54. Ho HK, Ha SY, Lam CK, et al. Alloimmunization in Hong Kong southern Chinese transfusion-dependent thalassemia patients. Blood 2001;97(12):3999–4000.

55. NIH, NHLBI. Evidence-based management of sickle cell disease: expert panel report. 2014. Available at: http://www.nhlbi.nih.gov/health-pro/guidelines/sickle-cell-disease-guidelines/. Accessed August 24, 2015.

56. Yawn BP, Buchanan GR, Afenyi-Annan AN, et al. Management of sickle cell dis-ease: summary of the 2014 evidence-based report by expert panel members. JAMA 2014;312(10):1033–48.

57. Vichinsky EP, Luban NL, Wright E, et al. Prospective RBC phenotype matching in a stroke-prevention trial in sickle cell anemia: a multicenter transfusion trial. Trans-fusion 2001;41(9):1086–92.

58. Lasalle-Williams M, Nuss R, Le T, et al. Extended red blood cell antigen matching for transfusions in sickle cell disease: a review of a 14-year experience from a sin-gle center (CME). Transfusion 2011;51(8):1732–9.

59. Tahhan HR, Holbrook CT, Braddy LR, et al. Antigen-matched donor blood in the transfusion management of patients with sickle-cell disease. Transfusion 1994; 34(7):562–9.

60. Webb J, Chou ST. Prospective antigen matching strategies fail to fit the model. Transfusion 2015;55(1):221–2.

61. Chou ST, Jackson T, Vege S, et al. High prevalence of red blood cell alloimmuni-zation in sickle cell disease despite transfusion from Rh-matched minority donors. Blood 2013;122(6):1062–71.

62. Denomme GA, Flegel WA. Applying molecular immunohematology discoveries to standards of practice in blood banks: now is the time. Transfusion 2008;48(11): 2461–75.

63. da Costa DC, Pellegrino J Jr, Guelsin GA, et al. Molecular matching of red blood cells is superior to serological matching in sickle cell disease patients. Rev Bras Hematol Hemoter 2013;35(1):35–8.

64. Singer ST, Wu V, Mignacca R, et al. Alloimmunization and erythrocyte autoimmu-nization in transfusion-dependent thalassemia patients of predominantly Asian descent. Blood 2000;96(10):3369–73.

65. el-Danasoury AS, Eissa DG, Abdo RM, et al. Red blood cell alloimmunization in transfusion-dependent Egyptian patients with thalassemia in a limited donor exposure program. Transfusion 2012;52(1):43–7.

66. Shirey RS, Boyd JS, Parwani AV, et al. Prophylactic antigen-matched donor blood for patients with warm autoantibodies: an algorithm for transfusion management. Transfusion 2002;42(11):1435–41.

67. Tormey CA, Stack G. The persistence and evanescence of blood group alloanti-bodies in men. Transfusion 2009;49(3):505–12.

68. Miller ST, Kim HY, Weiner DL, et al. Red blood cell alloimmunization in sickle cell disease: prevalence in 2010. Transfusion 2013;53(4):704–9.

69. FDA, US Department of Health and Human Services. Fatalities reported to the FDA following blood collection. 2012. Available at: http://www.fda.gov/BiologicsBloodVaccines/SafetyAvailability/ReportaProblem/TransfusionDonation Fatalities/default.htm. Accessed August 24, 2015.

Modifications to Blood Components

When to Use them and What is the Evidence?

Eric A. Gehrie, MD[a],*, Nancy M. Dunbar, MD[b,c]

KEYWORDS

- Red blood cells • Platelets • Transfusion medicine • Blood banking
- Transfusion reactions

KEY POINTS

- Blood components can be modified before issue to meet specific patient needs.
- Component modifications include leukoreduction, irradiation, volume reduction, splitting, and washing. With the exception of leukoreduction, which is nearly universally available in the United States and Canada, the other component modifications are time intensive.
- Transfusion medicine physicians can assist providers in selecting appropriate blood component modifications to meet patient needs.

TOPIC OVERVIEW INTRODUCTION

This article summarizes the benefits, drawbacks, and clinical considerations that should be factored into a decision to pursue specific blood component modifications.

LEUKOREDUCTION

Leukoreduction is the process of reducing the number of white blood cells (WBCs) in red blood cells (RBCs) and whole blood–derived or apheresis platelets (PLTs). In the United States and Canada, regulatory standards mandate that a leukoreduced blood component must contain fewer than 5×10^6 residual leukocytes ($<1 \times 10^6$ in Europe). Most leukoreduction in North America occurs during the blood component manufacturing process, either during apheresis collection or by using a specially designed filter that removes WBCs postcollection via adhesion.[1] These methods are commonly (and interchangeably) referred to as prestorage leukoreduction.

[a] Department of Laboratory Medicine, Yale University School of Medicine, 20 York Street, Blood Bank PS329C, New Haven, CT 06510-3206, USA; [b] Department of Pathology, Dartmouth-Hitchcock Medical Center, One Medical Center Drive, Lebanon, NH 03756-1000, USA; [c] Department of Medicine, Dartmouth-Hitchcock Medical Center, One Medical Center Drive, Lebanon, NH 03756-1000, USA
* Corresponding author.
E-mail address: eric.gehrie@yale.edu

Hematol Oncol Clin N Am 30 (2016) 653–663
http://dx.doi.org/10.1016/j.hoc.2016.01.007
0889-8588/16/$ – see front matter © 2016 Elsevier Inc. All rights reserved.

Alternatively, it is also possible to perform leukoreduction as the blood component is being infused into a patient (ie, poststorage leukoreduction or bedside leukoreduction), although this practice is uncommon.

Leukoreduction has been shown to decrease alloimmunization to human leukocyte antigens (HLAs), which may reduce the risk of refractoriness to PLT transfusion. The Trial to Reduce Alloimmunization to Platelets (TRAP) study showed that poststorage leukoreduction of PLTs reduced the rate of development of lymphocytotoxic antibodies as well as the incidence of PLT refractoriness in patients being treated for acute myeloid leukemia.[2] Specifically, it was estimated that 45% of patients receiving nonleukoreduced PLTs developed lymphocytotoxic antibodies, compared with 18% (P<.001) of patients receiving leukoreduced, pooled PLT units and 17% (P<.001) of patients receiving leukoreduced, apheresis PLT units. Furthermore, the TRAP study investigators estimated that 16% of patients transfused with nonleukoreduced PLTs developed PLT refractoriness, compared with 7% (P = .03) of patients receiving leukoreduced, pooled PLT units and 8% (P = .06) of patients transfused with leukoreduced, apheresis PLT units. There was no significant difference in the rate of PLT refractoriness when patients with a history of pregnancy were removed from the study groups, showing that patient-specific factors (in addition to product modifications) influence alloimmunization and refractoriness.[3] Consistent with the results of the TRAP trial, prestorage leukoreduction of PLTs was shown to reduce the incidence of PLT alloimmunization and PLT refractoriness, without altering the incidence of hemorrhage, among patients undergoing bone marrow transplantation in Canada.[4]

Leukoreduction is also generally thought to be equivalent to the use of cytomegalovirus (CMV) seronegative blood components in terms of prevention of transfusion-transmitted CMV infection (TT-CMV). In a prospective, randomized study of CMV-negative patients undergoing bone marrow transplant, the use of leukoreduced blood components, compared with blood components collected from CMV-seronegative donors, was not associated with a statistically significant increase in CMV infection or CMV disease from day 21 until day 100 posttransplant.[5] Although this study did report a statistically significant increase in CMV disease in early (before day 21) transplant recipients receiving leukoreduced transfusions (2.4% vs 0%, P = .03), another retrospective study found that there was no difference in the incidence of CMV viremia among bone marrow transplant patients receiving leukoreduced versus CMV-negative transfusions.[6] Therefore, leukoreduced blood is often referred to as CMV safe and blood donors in the United States are not required to be tested for CMV in order to donate.[7] However, for select populations at high risk for TT-CMV, hematologists may request leukoreduced blood components collected from CMV-seronegative donors.[8,9]

In addition, leukoreduction is also associated with a reduction in febrile nonhemolytic transfusion reactions (FNHTRs). These transfusion reactions are thought to be mediated, at least in part, by cytokines released from WBCs during storage. One retrospective study showed that the incidence of FNHTRs was reduced from 0.33% to 0.19% after instituting universal leukoreduction of RBCs (P<.001) and from 0.45% to 0.11% after instituting universal leukoreduction of PLTs (P<.001).[10] A similar retrospective study of RBC leukoreduction also showed a statistically significant reduction in FNHTRs from 0.37% before leukoreduction to 0.19% afterward (P = .0008).[11]

Prestorage leukoreduction of RBCs and PLTs is universal in Canada and is the predominant practice in the United States. Blood components labeled with ISBT (International Society of Blood Transfusion) 128–compliant labels have "Leukocytes Reduced" printed in the lower left corner of the label if the component has been prestorage leukoreduced.[12] Blood components that have undergone prestorage leukoreduction should be administered through a standard infusion set to exclude any clots or other debris that may have developed during storage. In contrast, because leukoreduction filters efficiently remove clots and debris as well as leukocytes, manufacturer instructions do not typically require the use of a filter in addition to a bedside leukoreduction set. Patients taking angiotensin-converting enzyme (ACE) inhibitors have been reported to have bradykinin-mediated hypotensive reactions, particularly during bedside leukoreduction procedures but also after infusion of prestorage leukoreduced blood components.[13,14] Leukoreduction is not considered to be an adequate alternative to irradiation for the prevention of transfusion-associated graft-versus-host disease (TA-GVHD). Hematopoietic stem cell products and granulocytes should never be leukoreduced.

Leukoreduction Summary

Benefits

- Reduces risk for HLA alloimmunization, PLT refractoriness, TT-CMV, and FNHTRs

Drawbacks

- Risk of hypotensive transfusion reactions (most commonly with bedside leukoreduction in patients treated with ACE inhibitors)

IRRADIATION

The sole purpose of irradiation of cellular blood components is the prevention of TA-GVHD. TA-GVHD is a clinical syndrome that occurs 2 days to 6 weeks following transfusion of a cellular blood component (RBCs, PLTs, and granulocytes) and is characterized by rash, diarrhea, fever, hepatomegaly, liver dysfunction, marrow aplasia, and pancytopenia.[15] This nearly uniformly fatal condition results from the engraftment of immunocompetent donor T lymphocytes that recognize the transfusion recipient as foreign and mount an immune attack on host tissues.[16]

Irradiation of cellular blood products prevents the proliferation of viable donor T lymphocytes. A dose of 25 Gy is required to completely inactivate T lymphocytes, although higher doses of radiation are required by regulatory authorities outside the United States.[17] In the United States, gamma irradiation is most commonly performed using a cesium-137 or cobalt-60 source, although use of X-irradiation is also an acceptable method.[18] New pathogen inactivation methods reduce T-lymphocyte viability and the use of these methods has replaced gamma irradiation of apheresis PLT products in some centers in Europe.[19–21] Although 1 pathogen inactivation method was recently approved by the US Food and Drug Administration (FDA), apheresis PLTs treated by this method are not yet widely available in North America. Although widespread availability of leukoreduced cellular blood products has been associated with a decrease in the incidence of TA-GVHD reported to government authorities,[22] leukoreduction is not considered to be an acceptable method to prevent TA-GVHD.

Prevention of TA-GVHD typically relies on recognition of patient risk factors and proper application of selective irradiation protocols. Irradiation is advised for all granulocyte transfusions and all liquid-stored RBC and PLT transfusions in at-risk patient populations. Recommendations for component irradiation are listed in **Box 1**. Irradiation is not required for previously frozen products such as plasma (including freeze-dried plasma), cryoprecipitate, and thawed deglycerolized RBCs.[18] Irradiation is absolutely contraindicated for hematopoietic progenitor cells.

Box 1
Summary of indications for irradiated blood components[a]

Blood components requiring irradiation for all recipients, regardless of age or clinical status

- HLA-matched or HLA-selected PLTs
- Granulocytes
- Directed donations of PLTs or RBCs

At-risk populations when irradiated RBCs and PLTs are indicated

- Allogeneic marrow and/or peripheral blood stem cell transplant recipients:
  - From the time of initiation of conditioning chemotherapy
- Autologous marrow and/or peripheral blood stem cell transplant recipients:
  - Any transfusions within 7 days of bone marrow/stem cell harvest
  - From the time of initiation of conditioning chemotherapy
- Patients with Hodgkin disease (any stage of disease)
- Patients with known or suspected congenital immunodeficiency affecting T lymphocytes
- Patients treated with purine analogues or purine antagonists; for example, fludarabine, cladribine, clofarabine, bendamustine, mercaptopurine pentostatin/deoxycoformycin, thioguanine
- Patients receiving bendamustine, alemtuzumab or anti-thymocyte globulin

At-risk pediatric populations when irradiated RBCs and PLTs are indicated:

- Fetus receiving an intrauterine transfusion
- Neonatal status (age<4 months), including neonatal exchange transfusions

[a] Institutions may opt to provide irradiated components for longer periods than recommended in this box; the decision to provide continued irradiated blood components may be made on a case-by-case basis with consideration of factors such as the type of transplant and the underlying disorder.

AABB standards require that cellular components be irradiated when the patient is at risk for TA-GVHD; when the donor of the blood component is a blood relative of the recipient, or when the donor is selected for HLA compatibility.[23] Application of universal irradiation of cellular blood products would effectively prevent all cases of TA-GVHD.

TA-GVHD is a rare complication of blood product transfusion. Since 2011 there have been 2 transfusion-related fatalities (1 in 2010, 1 in 2011) attributed to TA-GVHD reported to the FDA.[24] In 2011, only 13.4% of all cellular components transfused in the United States were irradiated.[25] This low percentage reflects the use of selective irradiation protocols in many centers.[26] Reasons for a selective approach include the substantial costs associated with purchasing and maintaining an irradiator, the limited throughput of typical irradiators, the cost of blood bank technical staff time, decreased shelf life (by up to 2 weeks) of irradiated RBCs, and security requirements associated with the source of radiation.[27] Irradiation is also associated with RBC membrane damage and increased supernatant potassium levels. Irradiated RBCs may pose increased risk for hyperkalemia in neonates, patients with renal dysfunction, and massive transfusion recipients.[28,29] Irradiation does not cause any known adverse effects to PLTs and does not require changes to the expiration date of the product. Recent reports are conflicting as to the impact of PLT irradiation on the efficacy of PLT transfusion.[30,31]

To avoid some of these drawbacks, many centers in the United States restrict the availability of irradiated RBCs to specific patient populations that are thought to be at greatest risk of TA-GVHD (see **Box 1**). Although potentially efficient, this practice also has several drawbacks. First, a patient who is at risk for TA-GVHD could be transfused with nonirradiated RBCs unless the person ordering blood products or the blood bank recognizes the risk for TA-GVHD. In busy hospitals, it is an operational challenge to screen every order for RBCs for TA-GVHD risk, and patients who ideally should receive irradiated RBCs may inadvertently end up receiving nonirradiated RBCs.[22,26]

In addition, although immunosuppression is thought to be the main risk factor for TA-GVHD in North America, there are multiple case reports of TA-GVHD occurring in immunocompetent patients for whom irradiation is not typically indicated.[16,32,33] Although uncommon, TA-GVHD in immunocompetent patients results from unidirectional tolerance toward a shared HLA haplotype between the HLA-heterozygous transfusion recipient and an HLA-homozygous blood component donor (**Fig. 1**). In the United States, based on population HLA haplotype frequencies, the predicted incidence of TA-GVHD is 1 in 17,700 to 1 in 39,000 if unidirectional tolerance is the sole determinant.[34] This risk increases significantly for recipients of blood from a family member.[35]

Irradiation Summary

Benefits

- Prevents TA-GVHD

Drawbacks

- Shortens unit expiration for irradiated RBCs by up to 2 weeks

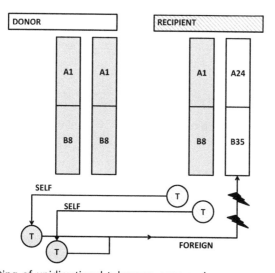

Fig. 1. In the setting of unidirectional tolerance, even an immunocompetent transfusion recipient from an HLA-homozygous donor is unable to recognize the transfused lymphocytes as foreign. However, because of the difference in HLA expression, the transfused lymphocytes recognize host tissues as foreign and mount an immune attack. Rectangles containing HLA antigens represent tissue. T, T lymphocytes.

- Increases risk for posttransfusion hyperkalemia in select populations because of increased supernatant potassium levels in stored irradiated RBCs
- Can delay immediate provision of blood components

VOLUME REDUCTION

Transfusion contributes significantly to the intravascular volume of the recipient. In many situations, transfusion recipients are able to compensate for such increases in intravascular volume because either (1) they are volume depleted because of bleeding, or (2) renal function is adequate to process and eliminate intravascular volume. However, if patients are unable to adequately compensate for transfusion-related increases in intravascular volume, serious adverse transfusion-related events, such as transfusion-associated circulatory overload or transfusion-associated dyspnea, may result.

Transfusions must be started before unit expiration and completed within 4 hours of issue from the blood bank.[36] In patients with diminished renal or cardiac function, or who already have volume overload, transfusing a unit of PLTs (typically 250 mL) or RBCs (typically 350 mL) over 4 hours may not be advisable. In these scenarios, the blood bank may volume reduce the component before issue to decrease risk for volume overload.

Volume reduction is feasible for RBCs and PLTs because these components contain cells suspended in a supernatant solution. For RBCs, the supernatant is predominantly an additive solution with a small amount of residual plasma. For PLTs, the supernatant solution is predominantly plasma or platelet additive solution. For volume-sensitive patients who require transfusion with RBCs or PLTs but are sensitive to volume, the supernatant solution can be removed before issue through unit centrifugation to isolate the cellular fraction. Volume reduction is typically performed immediately before unit issue. If volume-reduced RBCs or PLTs are administered to pediatric patients based on weight-based dosing (eg, 10–15 mL/kg), then the increased concentration of the volume-reduced unit should be taken into consideration in the determination of the appropriate dose. Consultation with a transfusion medicine physician is recommended before requesting volume reduction.

Volume Reduction Summary

Benefits

- Decreases volume to the patient

Drawbacks

- Delays availability of blood component
- Not available for plasma and cryoprecipitate

SPLITTING

For acellular products, such as plasma or cryoprecipitate, volume reduction cannot be performed. However, using a sterile docking device, units of plasma can be split into aliquots in the blood bank and issued separately to the hospital ward. Each aliquot of the split unit can be safely administered for 4 hours after issue, allowing slower infusion of the plasma product in patients who are at high risk for volume overload. RBCs and PLTs can also be split into aliquots in the blood bank. Cryoprecipitate is not typically split because it is stored in a frozen state and, unlike fresh frozen plasma, which expires 24 hours after thawing, cryoprecipitate expires 4 to 6 hours after thawing, making the logistics of slowly infusing smaller aliquots of cryoprecipitate challenging. In addition, a full dose of cryoprecipitate is typically only 100 to 150 mL. To accommodate small doses of cryoprecipitate (usually used for pediatric patients), many blood banks store small packets of cryoprecipitate, with each packet containing 10 to 15 mL. These packets can be thawed individually and infused as needed. Consultation with a transfusion medicine physician is recommended before requesting splitting.

Splitting Summary

Benefits

- Allows slow, gentle transfusion in patients at risk for fluid overload

Drawbacks

- Delays availability of blood component, although typically less so compared with volume reduction

WASHING

Washing of cellular components (RBCs and PLTs) replaces the plasma supernatant with saline. Washing is most commonly performed to decrease levels of plasma proteins in the transfused component for patients with a history of severe allergic transfusion reactions.[37] Washing may be also used to remove immunoglobulin A (IgA) in cellular components transfused to IgA-deficient recipients at risk for anaphylactic transfusion reactions caused by IgA antibodies; such an approach is typically adopted when components from IgA-deficient donors are unavailable.[38] In addition, washing of cellular blood components (and avoidance of plasma products) is recommended in patients with pneumococcal hemolytic uremic syndrome or other conditions in which T-antigen exposure is present.[39]

In addition to a reduction in levels of plasma proteins and antibodies to the T antigen, washing decreases levels of accumulated cytokines, potassium, and free hemoglobin in cellular components. A recent case report describes the successful application of washing to prevent recurrent acute hypotensive transfusion reactions attributed to vasodilators present in the plasma supernatant.[40]

Washing is accomplished by automated or manual methods through the addition and removal of 1 to 2 L of sterile normal saline, leaving sufficient saline behind to approximate a hematocrit of 50% to 80% for RBCs and a volume sufficient to maintain optimal storage conditions for PLTs.[41] Approximately 15% of the total hemoglobin and 33% of the PLT yield may be lost during the washing procedure.[42,43] Washing cannot be performed for plasma or cryoprecipitate.

Washing of cellular products has drawbacks. RBCs may experience shear stress, leading to increased fragility and plasma-free hemoglobin levels.[44] Recipients of washed PLTs show diminished PLT recovery and survival and may require more frequent PLT transfusions.[42] PLT washing is also associated with PLT activation and decreased aggregation.[45] The washing process is time consuming for the laboratory and may delay the availability of blood components. Washing removes anticoagulant-preservative solutions and may increase risk for bacterial contamination. RBCs must be transfused within 24 hours after washing and PLTs within 4 hours after washing. Consultation with a transfusion medicine physician is recommended before requesting washing.

Table 1
Applicability of modifications to various blood components

Component	Leukoreduction	Irradiation	Volume Reduction	Split	Washing
RBCs	Yes	Yes	Yes	Yes	Yes
Plasma[a]	Yes[b]	No	No	Yes	No
PLTs	Yes	Yes	Yes	Yes	Yes
Cryoprecipitate	NA	No	No	Yes[c]	No
Granulocytes	Never	Always	Yes[c]	Yes[c]	No

Abbreviation: NA, not applicable.
 [a] Includes fresh frozen plasma, thawed plasma, liquid plasma, plasma frozen within 24 hours, and cryoprecipitate-poor plasma.
 [b] Plasma is generally considered to be an acellular product, but bedside leukoreduction filters are commercially available.
 [c] Technically possible, but generally not a feasible practice given the shelf life.

Washing Summary

Benefits

- Decrease risk for severe allergic transfusion reactions
- Removal of antibodies to the T antigen

Drawbacks

- Delays availability of blood component
- Shortens product expiration
- Not available for plasma and cryoprecipitate
- May be damaging to RBCs and PLTs

SUMMARY

Leukoreduction, irradiation, volume reduction, splitting, and washing of select blood components may be performed by the hospital blood bank for certain clinical indications. The applicability of these modifications to commonly available blood components is summarized in **Table 1**. The modifications discussed in this article may not be available at all hospitals, are associated with increased costs, and may delay the availability of the blood component because of the additional time required for some modification steps. Consultation with a transfusion medicine physician is recommended before requesting volume reduction, splitting, or washing.

REFERENCES

1. Dzik S. Leukodepletion blood filters: filter design and mechanisms of leukocyte removal. Transfus Med Rev 1993;7(2):65–77.
2. Leukocyte reduction and ultraviolet B irradiation of platelets to prevent alloimmunization and refractoriness to platelet transfusions. The Trial to Reduce Alloimmunization to Platelets study group. N Engl J Med 1997;337(26):1861–9.
3. Gehrie EA, Tormey CA. The influence of clinical and biological factors on transfusion-associated non-ABO antigen alloimmunization: responders, hyperresponders, and non-responders. Transfus Med Hemother 2014;41(6):420–9.
4. Seftel MD, Growe GH, Petraszko T, et al. Universal prestorage leukoreduction in Canada decreases platelet alloimmunization and refractoriness. Blood 2004; 103(1):333–9.

5. Bowden RA, Slichter SJ, Sayers M, et al. A comparison of filtered leukocyte-reduced and cytomegalovirus (CMV) seronegative blood products for the prevention of transfusion-associated CMV infection after marrow transplant. Blood 1995;86(9):3598–603.

6. Kekre N, Tokessy M, Mallick R, et al. Is cytomegalovirus testing of blood products still needed for hematopoietic stem cell transplant recipients in the era of universal leukoreduction? Biol Blood Marrow Transplant 2013;19(12):1719–24.

7. Narvios AB, de Lima M, Shah H, et al. Transfusion of leukoreduced cellular blood components from cytomegalovirus-unscreened donors in allogeneic hematopoietic transplant recipients: analysis of 72 recipients. Bone Marrow Transplant 2005;36(6):499–501.

8. Smith D, Lu Q, Yuan S, et al. Survey of current practice for prevention of transfusion-transmitted cytomegalovirus in the United States: leucoreduction vs. cytomegalovirus-seronegative. Vox Sang 2010;98(1):29–36.

9. Nichols WG, Price TH, Gooley T, et al. Transfusion-transmitted cytomegalovirus infection after receipt of leukoreduced blood products. Blood 2003;101(10): 4195–200.

10. Yazer MH, Podlosky L, Clarke G, et al. The effect of prestorage WBC reduction on the rates of febrile nonhemolytic transfusion reactions to platelet concentrates and RBC. Transfusion 2004;44(1):10–5.

11. King KE, Shirey RS, Thoman SK, et al. Universal leukoreduction decreases the incidence of febrile nonhemolytic transfusion reactions to RBCs. Transfusion 2004;44(1):25–9.

12. ISBT 128 for blood components: an introduction. In: Ashford P, editor. 3rd edition. San Bernardino (CA): ICCBBA; 2014. Available at: https://iccbba.org/uploads/02/ce/02cedb115f9f9f53a574808e48712bae/IN-003-ISBT-128-for-Blood-Components-An-Introduction-v3.pdf. Accessed February 13, 2016.

13. Quillen K. Hypotensive transfusion reactions in patients taking angiotensin-converting-enzyme inhibitors. N Engl J Med 2000;343(19):1422–3.

14. Arnold DM, Molinaro G, Warkentin TE, et al. Hypotensive transfusion reactions can occur with blood products that are leukoreduced before storage. Transfusion 2004;44(9):1361–6.

15. National Healthcare Safety Network Biovigilance component Hemovigilance module surveillance protocol. Available at: http://www.cdc.gov/nhsn/PDFs/Biovigilance/BV-HV-protocol-current.pdf. Accessed February 13, 2016.

16. Jawa RS, Young DH, Stothert JC, et al. Transfusion-associated graft versus host disease in the immunocompetent patient: an ongoing problem. J Intensive Care Med 2015;30(3):123–30.

17. Pelszynski MM, Moroff G, Luban NL, et al. Effect of gamma irradiation of red blood cell units on T-cell inactivation as assessed by limiting dilution analysis: implications for preventing transfusion-associated graft-versus-host disease. Blood 1994;83(6):1683–9.

18. Treleaven J, Gennery A, Marsh J, et al. Guidelines on the use of irradiated blood components prepared by the British Committee for Standards in Haematology Blood Transfusion Task Force. Br J Haematol 2011;152(1):35–51.

19. Cazenave JP, Isola H, Waller C, et al. Use of additive solutions and pathogen inactivation treatment of platelet components in a regional blood center: impact on patient outcomes and component utilization during a 3-year period. Transfusion 2011;51(3):622–9.

20. Fast LD, Nevola M, Tavares J, et al. Treatment of whole blood with riboflavin plus ultraviolet light, an alternative to gamma irradiation in the prevention of

transfusion-associated graft-versus-host disease? Transfusion 2013;53(2):
373–81.

21. Schlenke P. Pathogen inactivation technologies for cellular blood components: an update. Transfus Med Hemother 2014;41(4):309–25.

22. Bolton-Maggs PHB, Chapman C, Mistry H. Continued absence of transfusion-associated graft versus host disease despite failures to provide irradiated products to patients at risk - more than a decade of data from SHOT. Br J Haematol 2012;157(Suppl 1):3.

23. Standards for blood banks and transfusion services. 29th edition. Bethesda (MD): AABB; 2014.

24. Fatalities reported to FDA following blood collection and transfusion: annual summary for fiscal year 2013. Available at: http://www.fda.gov/Biologics BloodVaccines/SafetyAvailability/ReportaProblem/TransfusionDonationFatalities/ ucm391574.htm. Accessed February 13, 2016.

25. Whitaker BI, Hinkins S. 2011 National Blood Collection and Utilization Survey. 2011. Available at: http://www.hhs.gov/ash/bloodsafety/2011-nbcus.pdf. Accessed February 13, 2016.

26. Ness PM, Lipton KS. Selective transfusion protocols: errors and accidents waiting to happen. Transfusion 2001;41(5):713–5.

27. Mintz PD, Wehrli G. Irradiation eradication and pathogen reduction. Ceasing cesium irradiation of blood products. Bone Marrow Transplant 2009;44(4): 205–11.

28. Vraets A, Lin Y, Callum JL. Transfusion-associated hyperkalemia. Transfus Med Rev 2011;25(3):184–96.

29. Lee AC, Reduque LL, Luban NL, et al. Transfusion-associated hyperkalemic cardiac arrest in pediatric patients receiving massive transfusion. Transfusion 2014; 54(1):244–54.

30. Zhu M, Xu W, Wang BL, et al. Hemostatic function and transfusion efficacy of apheresis platelet concentrates treated with gamma irradiation in use for thrombocytopenic patients. Transfus Med Hemother 2014;41(3):189–96.

31. Julmy F, Ammann RA, Fontana S, et al. Transfusion efficacy of apheresis platelet concentrates irradiated at the day of transfusion is significantly superior compared to platelets irradiated in advance. Transfus Med Hemother 2014; 41(3):176–81.

32. Agbaht K, Altintas ND, Topeli A, et al. Transfusion-associated graft-versus-host disease in immunocompetent patients: case series and review of the literature. Transfusion 2007;47(8):1405–11.

33. O'Brien KL, Pereira SE, Wagner J, et al. Transfusion-associated graft-versus-host disease in a liver transplant recipient: an unusual presentation and review of the literature. Transfusion 2013;53(1):174–80.

34. Wagner FF, Flegel WA. Transfusion-associated graft-versus-host disease: risk due to homozygous HLA haplotypes. Transfusion 1995;35(4):284–91.

35. Ohto H, Yasuda H, Noguchi M, et al. Risk of transfusion-associated graft-versus-host disease as a result of directed donations from relatives. Transfusion 1992; 32(7):691–3.

36. Circular of information for the use of human blood and blood components. AABB, American Red Cross, America's Blood Centers, and the Armed Services Blood Program; 2014. Available at: http://www.aabb.org/tm/coi/Documents/coi1113. pdf. Accessed February 13, 2016.

37. Tobian AA, Savage WJ, Tisch DJ, et al. Prevention of allergic transfusion reactions to platelets and red blood cells through plasma reduction. Transfusion 2011;51(8):1676–83.

38. Sandler SG. How I manage patients suspected of having had an IgA anaphylactic transfusion reaction. Transfusion 2006;46(1):10–3.

39. Cochran JB, Panzarino VM, Maes LY, et al. *Pneumococcus*-induced T-antigen activation in hemolytic uremic syndrome and anemia. Pediatr Nephrol 2004; 19(3):317–21.

40. Crews WS Jr, Kay JK, Herman JH. Washed RBCs prevent recurrent acute hypotensive transfusion reactions. Am J Clin Pathol 2014;141(2):285–7.

41. Hansen A, Yi QL, Acker JP. Quality of red blood cells washed using the ACP 215 cell processor: assessment of optimal pre- and postwash storage times and conditions. Transfusion 2013;53(8):1772–9.

42. Karafin M, Fuller AK, Savage WJ, et al. The impact of apheresis platelet manipulation on corrected count increment. Transfusion 2012;52(6):1221–7.

43. Weisbach V, Riego W, Strasser E, et al. The in vitro quality of washed, prestorage leucocyte-depleted red blood cell concentrates. Vox Sang 2004;87(1):19–26.

44. Harm SK, Raval JS, Cramer J, et al. Haemolysis and sublethal injury of RBCs after routine blood bank manipulations. Transfus Med 2012;22(3):181–5.

45. Veeraputhiran M, Ware J, Dent J, et al. A comparison of washed and volume-reduced platelets with respect to platelet activation, aggregation, and plasma protein removal. Transfusion 2011;51(5):1030–6.

Management of the Platelet Refractory Patient

Stefanie K. Forest, MD, PhD[a], Eldad A. Hod, MD[b],*

KEYWORDS

- Platelet • Transfusion • Refractoriness • HLA • HPA • Alloimmunization

KEY POINTS

- Platelet refractoriness is defined as an inadequate response to platelet transfusions and is diagnosed by a corrected count increment of less than 5×10^9/L after 2 sequential transfusions.
- Nonimmune causes are the most likely and the first that should be explored in the diagnosis of platelet refractoriness.
- Immune-mediated platelet refractoriness is cause by antibodies to human leukocyte antigens (HLAs) and/or human platelet antigens.
- If antibodies are identified, there are 3 strategies for identifying compatible platelet units: HLA matching, crossmatching, and antibody specificity prediction.

INTRODUCTION

Platelets play an integral role in the maintenance of hemostasis by adhering to sites of vascular injury and forming a platelet plug. Platelets are anucleate discoid-shaped cells, 3 to 5 μm in diameter by 0.5 μm in depth, derived from bone marrow megakaryocytes. In healthy individuals, they circulate at a level of 150×10^9 to 400×10^9 platelets per liter. Thrombocytopenia can lead to bleeding symptoms ranging from petechiae and simple bruising to intracranial hemorrhage, pulmonary hemorrhage, and death. Low platelet counts are the result of either decreased production of platelets from factors adversely affecting megakaryocyte production in the bone marrow or increased destruction of platelets.[1]

Platelet transfusions became routinely available in the 1970s when Murphy and Gardner[3] showed that platelets could be stored at 22°C, for up to 3 days and still

Disclosure: The authors have nothing to disclose.
[a] Department of Pathology and Cell Biology, Columbia University Medical Center, New York-Presbyterian Hospital, 630 West 168th Street, VC 14-239, New York, NY 10032, USA;
[b] Department of Pathology and Cell Biology, Columbia University Medical Center, New York-Presbyterian Hospital, 630 West 168th Street, P&S 14-434, New York, NY 10032, USA
* Corresponding author.
E-mail address: eh2217@cumc.columbia.edu

Hematol Oncol Clin N Am 30 (2016) 665–677
http://dx.doi.org/10.1016/j.hoc.2016.01.008
0889-8588/16/$ – see front matter © 2016 Elsevier Inc. All rights reserved.

hemonc.theclinics.com

maintain their function.[2,3] Platelet transfusions are now commonly used for both qualitative and quantitative platelet defects. Current guidelines recommend prophylactic platelet transfusions at a threshold of less than or equal to 10×10^9 platelets per liter.[4] With current advances in oncologic therapies as well as the use of hematopoietic stem cell transplantation, more patients develop severe hypoproliferative thrombocytopenia for longer durations than were previously seen and this often requires platelet transfusion support.[4] The availability of effective platelet transfusions has decreased mortality from bleeding complications in these patient populations.[5] In some patients, the observed platelet increment following transfusion is significantly less than the expected increment. Although these inadequate responses to platelet transfusions (ie, platelet refractoriness) have decreased with increased usage of leukoreduced products, they still occur and are of serious concern to both clinicians and the transfusion services supporting the special transfusion needs of these patients.

DEFINITION OF PLATELET REFRACTORINESS

Platelet refractoriness can be simply defined as a posttransfusion platelet increment that is less than expected. The Trial to Reduce Alloimmunization to Platelets (TRAP) study[6] defined platelet refractoriness as a corrected count increment (CCI) (Box 1) of less than 5×10^9/L after 2 sequential transfusions, using ABO-compatible platelets, at least 1 of which had been stored for no more than 48 hours, with a posttransfusion platelet count obtained within an hour after transfusion. This definition has been generally accepted by the American Society of Clinical Oncology.[7] The CCI formula takes both the number of platelets transfused and the patient's body surface area into account. Furthermore, the timing of the posttransfusion platelet count is important for the interpretation of the CCI. A 1-hour posttransfusion count is preferred because it requires at least 1 hour to reach intravascular equilibrium after transfusion.[8] However, in a busy hospital, a 1-hour posttransfusion platelet count can be difficult to obtain, and therefore some clinicians have advocated using a 10-minute posttransfusion count.[9] The timing of the posttransfusion platelet count can be suggestive of the cause of refractoriness; a low CCI before 1 hour after transfusion is suggestive of immune causes, whereas a reduced CCI at 18 to 24 hours following a normal CCI at 1 hour is more suggestive of increased platelet consumption from other nonimmune clinical factors.[10] It is currently recommended that the following criteria be used to determine platelet refractoriness[11]: A 10-minute to 1-hour posttransfusion CCI of less than 5×10^9/L, observed on at least 2 sequential occasions, using ABO-identical freshest available platelets.

Box 1
CCI calculation

$$CCI^a = \frac{\text{posttransfusion platelet count} - \text{pretransfusion platelet count } (/L) \times BSA \ (m^2)^b}{\text{platelets transfused } (10^{11})^c}$$

Abbreviation: BSA, body surface area.

[a] For example, using a BSA of 2.0 m^2, an absolute platelet increment of less than 10×10^9/L after administration of an apheresis unit of platelets is suspect for refractoriness (CCI<5.0 × 10^9/L).

[b] Average adult BSA = 2.0 m^2.

[c] Platelets transfused = approximately 4×10^{11} platelets in apheresis unit, 0.7×10^{11} for each random donor platelet concentrate.

CAUSE

Platelet refractoriness can have both immune and nonimmune causes (**Boxes 2 and 3**). Although the nonimmune causes are more likely to be responsible for a poor response to a platelet transfusion, there is little a transfusion service can do, other than recommending treating the underlying disorder, to improve the outcome of transfusion in these cases. Thus, the discussion focuses on the immune causes of platelet refractoriness.

The most common immune causes of platelet refractoriness are antibodies to human leukocyte antigens (HLAs) and/or human platelet antigens (HPAs), with anti-HLA antibodies more commonly responsible. The presence of these antibodies can be caused by prior exposure from pregnancy, transfusions, and/or transplantation.

The HLA system arises from the major histocompatibility complex that encodes polymorphic cell-surface proteins important for antigen presentation. Platelets express HLA class I antigens. HLA class I antigens consist of HLA-A, HLA-B, and HLA-C; HLA-A and HLA-B antigens predominate on platelets and are considered most relevant for platelet refractoriness.[12] However, HLA-C antigens have also been reported to cause platelet refractoriness.[13] Primary immunization against HLAs is caused by contaminating leukocytes in the platelet product[14] and reducing contaminating leukocytes in blood products by filtration or ultraviolet B irradiation reduces the development of lymphocytotoxic antibodies and alloimmune platelet refractoriness to transfusions compared with untreated pooled platelet concentrates from random donors.[6]

There are several platelet-specific antigens that have been characterized; however, only 5 of them are known to be polymorphic, leading to alloimmunization and platelet refractoriness: GPIa, GPIb, GPIIb, GPIIIA, and CD109.[12] There are significant differences in the prevalence of the HPA polymorphisms in various populations, and patients become alloimmunized to these antigens through transfusions and pregnancy. Leukoreduction does not affect the incidence of platelet-specific antibodies, which varies from 2% to 11%.[6,15,16] Furthermore, platelet-specific antibodies are generally not associated with a statistically significant reduction in CCI.[6,17] Although case reports describe platelet-specific antibodies causing refractoriness to transfusion, these cases are usually confounded by concurrent anti-HLA antibodies.[18]

Box 2
Nonimmune causes of platelet refractoriness

Sepsis

Fever

Splenomegaly

Disseminated intravascular coagulation

Medications[a]

Graft-versus-host disease

Bleeding

Venoocclusive disease[b]

  [a] See **Box 3** for list of medications.
  [b] Controversial.[7]

Box 3
Partial list of medications with documentation supporting an association with drug-induced thrombocytopenia or with the formation of drug-dependent platelet antibodies

Infectious disease agents

Ampicillin

Amoxicillin

Cephalosporins

Ciprofloxacin/levofloxacin

Linezolid

Metronidazole

Nafcillin

Penicillin

Piperacillin/tazobactam

Rifampin

Sulfonamides

Vancomycin

Amphotericin

Trimethoprim/sulfamethoxazole

Suramin

Ethambutol

Histamine-receptor antagonists

Cimetidine

Famotidine

Ranitidine

Analgesics

Acetaminophen

Diclofenac

Fentanyl

Ibuprofen

Naproxen

Salicylates

Chemotherapeutics and immunosuppressants

Bleomycin

Cyclosporine

Oxaliplatin

Fludarabine

Rituximab

Irinotecan

Antithrombotics

Clopidogrel/ticlopidine

GPIIb/GPIIIa antagonists

Heparin

Cinchona alkaloids

Quinine

Quinidine

Sedatives and anticonvulsant agents

Carbamazepine

Phenytoin

Valproic acid

Cholesterol management

Simvastatin

Psychiatric medications

Mirtazapine

Haloperidol

Adapted from Refs.[40–42]; and George JN. Platelets on the web: drug-induced thrombocytopenia. Available at: http://www.ouhsc.edu/platelets/ditp.html. Accessed March 25, 2016.

Most patients who have HLA antibodies do not develop platelet refractoriness. In the TRAP study, 45% of the control group developed anti-HLA antibodies, but only 13% developed platelet refractoriness. A dose-response relationship between the number of platelets transfused and the incidence of alloimmunization is also not observed.[19,20] In the TRAP trial, there was no difference in lymphocytotoxic antibodies or platelet refractoriness following transfusion of platelets obtained by apheresis from a single random donor compared with pooled platelet concentrates from random donors, which is surprising considering there is exposure to more donor HLA and HPA in pooled platelet concentrates.[6] This finding suggests that alloimmunization and refractoriness are complicated processes with unknown modifying factors determining whether an individual will become alloimmunized and, subsequently, whether this alloimmunization will cause refractoriness to transfusion.[7]

TRANSFUSION SERVICE FACTORS

In addition to the immune causes of platelet refractoriness, transfusion service factors, such as the storage of the platelet product and ABO compatibility, also affect platelet increments. Platelets show variable expression of ABH antigens on their surface; these antigens are both intrinsic to the platelet membrane and passively adsorbed from plasma.[21] Thus, recipient ABO antibodies can increase the clearance of transfused incompatible platelets.[22] Furthermore, platelets can be stored at room temperature for 5 days before transfusion. In vitro markers of platelet quality decline by day 5 of storage[23] and platelet age significantly affects CCI, with platelets stored for less than 48 hours resulting in a significantly improved platelet increment at both 1 hour and 18 to 24 hours following transfusion.[24] Thus, the CCI can be improved by using ABO-compatible and fresh platelets (ie, stored for less than 48 hours)[24] and these factors must be considered when assessing patients for platelet refractoriness and for providing optimal care.

INCIDENCE

Based on the TRAP study, in a study population of patients with acute myeloid leukemia (AML) receiving standard induction chemotherapy, 16% of patients receiving non-leukodepleted products met the criteria for refractoriness, as opposed to 7% to 10% of patients receiving leukodepleted products.[6] Depending on the study population and the definition of refractoriness, the incidence of refractoriness in hematology/oncology patients varies from 7% to 34%.[6,25,26] It is estimated that approximately two-thirds of refractory episodes have nonalloimmune causes, with another 20% having a combination of both alloimmune and nonalloimmune causes.[25,27]

LABORATORY DIAGNOSIS OF IMMUNE-MEDIATED PLATELET REFRACTORINESS

There are several laboratory tests available to determine whether a patient with platelet refractoriness has anti-HLA and/or anti-HPA antibodies. However, there is no consensus regarding which test is ideal for diagnosing refractoriness.[28] Some assays may be too sensitive, identifying weak HLA antibodies that do not predict platelet refractoriness. Cell-based cytotoxicity assays may better predict platelet refractoriness; however, these tests are more cumbersome than the more automated techniques.[12] Thus, the results of platelet refractoriness testing should be interpreted in conjunction with the clinical picture and, in the absence of a gold standard test, a change in transfusion management should only be pursued if both clinical and laboratory evidence suggest the presence of true immune-mediated platelet refractoriness.

MANAGEMENT

Several factors should be considered in the management of patients with platelet refractoriness. Potential nonimmune causes (see **Boxes 2** and **3**) should be assessed and, if possible, corrected and controlled to see whether the response to platelet transfusions is improved. ABO-matched and freshest available platelets should be used when possible. An immune cause of platelet refractoriness should be evaluated by determining the presence of HLA and HPA antibodies. If antibodies are identified, there are 3 strategies (**Table 1**) for identifying compatible platelet units:

- HLA matching
- Crossmatching
- Antibody specificity prediction

Other strategies for managing thrombocytopenic refractory patients have generally met with limited success (**Table 2**). For instance, immune thrombocytopenic purpura has been treated with splenectomy and anti-Rh(D); however, evidence does not support their use in platelet refractory recipients. These alternative strategies have been reported mainly in small uncontrolled studies or case reports and no clear-cut recommendations can be made regarding these therapies.[10]

HUMAN LEUKOCYTE ANTIGEN MATCHING

One technique for providing platelets for patients with platelet refractoriness and HLA antibodies is to provide HLA-matched platelets. Once the recipient's HLA type is known, platelets from a donor with identical, or a similar, HLA type (see **Table 3** for the grading system used to assess the degree of matching) should be provided. These HLA-matched platelets should improve platelet count increments if the HLA antibodies are responsible for refractoriness.[29] Thus, a CCI should be calculated following

Table 1
Methods for managing immune-mediated platelet refractoriness

	HLA Matched	Crossmatched	Antibody Specificity Prediction
Method	HLA type the patient and provide platelets collected from an HLA-matched donor	Combine donor platelets with patient's serum to determine crossmatch compatibility	Identify HLA antibodies in patient and then provide platelets without those specific HLAs
Pros	Prevents future alloimmunization if high-grade match	• Useful for anti-HPA and anti-HLA • Rapid availability • HLA typing not required	• Larger donor pool • Patient HLA typing not required
Cons	• Not useful for anti-HPA • Patient and donor HLA typing required • Must recruit HLA-matched donors • Limited donor pool for rare HLA types	• Difficult to find suitable crossmatch in highly sensitized patients • Risk of alloimmunization against mismatched donor HLAs • Frequent crossmatching necessary	• Not useful for anti-HPA • Potential risk of alloimmunization against mismatched donor HLAs • Must type donor HLA

the provision of HLA-matched platelets to determine whether to continue with this management.

Because immune-mediated platelet refractoriness is typically caused by antibodies to the HLA class I, HLA-A and HLA-B antigens, platelets are only matched for these loci.[30] In addition, the better the HLA match between donor and recipient, the better the outcome. Thus, there is good correlation between the match grade (see **Table 3**) and the CCI after transfusion; A or BU matches are associated with the most successful platelet transfusions, but are still associated with a failure rate of up to 20%.[31] In a more recent study, 30% of HLA-selected platelet transfusions (A, B1U, or B1X match grade) compared with 12% of random-donor transfusions gave a satisfactory response to transfusion, defined as a CCI of more than 5.0×10^9/L.[32] Although there were more satisfactory responses with HLA-selected platelets compared with random-donor platelets, 70% of HLA-selected platelet transfusions did not give a satisfactory response. Furthermore, there was no significant difference in the 1-hour to 4-hour CCIs when comparing HLA-selected units with random-donor units.[32] Thus, although there is improvement in platelet responses with HLA-selected units, most HLA-selected platelet transfusions do not lead to a satisfactory CCI, possibly because of other clinical factors that contribute to platelet refractoriness.

One of the main issues with providing HLA-matched platelets is the availability of these products. Models developed to determine the donor pool size necessary to support a patient population at a given match grade suggest that a pool of up to 3000 donors is needed to meet the transfusion needs at an HLA match grade level of Bx or better.[33] In addition, for HLA-matched platelets, both the patient and the donor must be HLA typed. This requirement increases costs and leads to delays in providing HLA-matched platelets.

CROSSMATCHING

Another management strategy for providing platelets to patients with immune causes of refractoriness is to provide crossmatched platelets. These platelets are useful for

Table 2
Alternative management strategies

Treatment	Findings	Reference	Summary
Antifibrinolytics	Studies using epsilon-aminocaproic acid or tranexamic acid suggest decreased bleeding and need for platelet and red cell transfusions. No thromboembolic complications reported	43–46	Can be used as an adjunctive therapy in patients refractory to platelet transfusions
IVIG	Consensus recommendations for off-label use of intravenous IVIG states that, for patients with thrombocytopenia and refractoriness to platelet transfusions, evidence does not support routine use of IVIG. It may have some role in patients with severe thrombocytopenia of documented immune basis for whom other modalities are unsuccessful or contraindicated	47–49	This expensive treatment should not be used or considered as replacement for HLA-compatible platelets for alloimmunized patients
Splenectomy	No effect on posttransfusion CCI in alloimmunized patients	50	Not recommended
Anti-Rh(D)	In a randomized trial, anti-Rh(D) showed no effect on the rate of refractoriness or number of platelet concentrates required per day. Significantly increases the requirement for red cell transfusions	51	Not recommended
Protein A column	Small study using 10 refractory patients. Protein A column therapy was effective in improving platelet response in 6 patients; no follow-up study	52	Unclear evidence. Protein A columns unavailable at many institutions and have potential side effects
Massive platelet dose transfusion	In animal studies and 2 alloimmunized humans, infusion of a massive dose of platelets to absorb the alloantibodies led to significant improvement in subsequent platelet transfusions and in bleeding symptoms	53	Anecdotal evidence. May be considered for arresting hemorrhage in emergency situations when compatible platelets are unavailable

(continued on next page)

Table 2
(continued)

Treatment	Findings	Reference	Summary
Continuous slow platelet transfusion	Anecdotal success in 3 patients with AML and platelet refractoriness when platelet concentrate was infused slowly over 6 h	54	Anecdotal evidence. Small-dose frequent platelet transfusions may be helpful in maintaining vascular integrity despite lack of increase in posttransfusion platelet count
Activated factor VII	Anecdotal success in controlling bleeding in platelet refractory patients	55,56	Anecdotal evidence. There is concern for prothrombotic risk. May be considered for arresting hemorrhage in emergency situations

Abbreviation: IVIG, immunoglobulin.
Data from Refs.[43–56]

patients with anti-HLA and/or anti-HPA antibodies. There are several methods used for platelet crossmatching, but in general these involve incubating donor platelets with recipient plasma and testing for an interaction.[12] Crossmatching allows rapid and effective selection of donor platelets and can be performed in a few hours as opposed to the days it may take to test, schedule, and collect an appropriate HLA-matched donor.[34] Furthermore, these methods make it feasible for most blood centers to perform platelet crossmatching in large numbers and in a short time frame.[35]

A recent systematic review showed superior CCIs in patients who received crossmatch-compatible units compared with random or crossmatch-incompatible units, with a success rate ranging from 50% to 90%.[36] Using radiolabeled platelets, crossmatch-compatible platelets were shown to survive for 3.5 to 8.7 days, whereas incompatible platelets survived for only 0.1 to 2.4 days.[37] However, there seems to be little difference between the 1-hour CCI of crossmatched platelets compared with HLA-matched platelets[31]; thus, either approach is appropriate. Furthermore, a disadvantage of the platelet crossmatch is that the limited shelf life of platelets of 5 days demands frequent crossmatches for patients requiring long-term platelet support.[38] In addition, because of the possibility of a change in alloantibody reactivity,

Table 3
HLA match grade

Grade	Degree of Matching
A	All 4-HLA-A and HLA-B loci are identical
BU	Only 3 antigens detected in donor; all present in recipient Recipient cells do not possess HLA-A or HLA-B antigens that differ from donor because of homozygosity at HLA-A or HLA-B loci
BX	Three donor antigens identical to recipient One HLA-A or HLA-B incompatibility that is cross reactive
C	Three donor antigens identical to recipient One noncrossreactive antigen difference
D	Two or more noncrossreactive mismatches

crossmatches should be performed on a fresh sample drawn from the recipient every 72 hours.[7]

ANTIBODY SPECIFICITY PREDICTION

A third general strategy for managing alloimmunization is similar to the approach routinely used for red blood cell alloimmunization. In antibody specificity prediction (ASP), the specificity of the recipient's HLA antibodies is identified and then the patient is provided with platelets from donors lacking only those HLAs to which the patient has antibodies. Therefore, unlike the strategy of HLA matching, which matches recipient and donor HLA-A and HLA-B types, the ASP method does not require a full match; only the antigens to which the patient has alloantibodies are matched. This method increases the donor pool significantly. For example, among 7247 HLA-typed donors, for each HLA-alloimmunized patient a mean of 6 donors were HLA-A matched, 33 were HLA-BU matched, and 1426 were identified by ASP.[38] In an observational study of 114 refractory patients receiving 1621 platelet transfusions, and comparing platelets that were HLA matched, crossmatch compatible, chosen by ASP, or randomly selected, the mean platelet count increment was similar for the first 3 methods and was significantly better than for randomly selected platelet transfusions.[38]

SUMMARY OF RECOMMENDATIONS

Refractoriness to platelet transfusion is a complex process and poses a great challenge for the treatment of thrombocytopenic patients. The best platelet product to provide patients with platelet refractoriness is a challenging question with practical considerations of inventory management and cost. Fresh and ABO-matched platelet products are recommended where possible. In addition, it is helpful to use fresh and ABO-matched platelets in the diagnosis of platelet refractoriness to eliminate these potential variables as causes of refractoriness. Inventory management sometimes restricts the use of fresh ABO-matched platelets. Platelets have a short shelf life of 5 days and, in order to avoid waste, most blood banks have inventory management of last-in-first-out policies. Therefore, providing fresh platelets is a challenge.[39] The authors recommend freshest available platelets where possible, especially in assessing potential refractory patients.

After ruling out nonimmune causes of platelet refractoriness (see **Boxes 2** and **3**), the diagnosis of immune-mediated platelet refractoriness should be made by calculating 2 sequential 10-minute to 1-hour CCIs. If the CCI is less than $5 \times 10^9/L$[11] then a test for the presence of anti-HLA and anti-HPA antibodies should be performed. If the patient is found to have these antibodies, then there are 3 main approaches for the management of immune causes of platelet refractoriness. Each strategy (ie, HLA matching, crossmatching, and the ASP method) has advantages and disadvantages (see **Table 1**). They seem to offer similar results in terms of posttransfusion CCI.[38] However, there are no randomized clinical trials comparing the effectiveness of these methods on clinical outcomes.

It is recommended to assess the effectiveness of a chosen management strategy by determining the CCI for each platelet transfusion following the provision of matched platelets. Failure to achieve an appropriate CCI may be caused by the presence of nonimmune causes of platelet refractoriness, which should be treated before obtaining matched platelets. Clinicians have yet to fully understand the interplay of factors that affect the response to platelet transfusion or whether a patient will form an alloantibody to HLA or platelet antigens. Although there has been considerable progress in diagnosing, preventing, and managing immune-mediated refractoriness to platelet transfusion, the care of these patients can still be improved.

REFERENCES

1. Lochowicz AJ, Curtis BR. Clinical applications of platelet antibody and antigen testing. Lab Med 2011;42(11):687–92.
2. Blajchman MA. Platelet transfusions: an historical perspective. Hematology Am Soc Hematol Educ Program 2008;1:197.
3. Murphy S, Gardner FH. Effect of storage temperature on maintenance of platelet viability–deleterious effect of refrigerated storage. N Engl J Med 1969;280(20): 1094–8.
4. Nahirniak S, Slichter SJ, Tanael S, et al. Guidance on platelet transfusion for patients with hypoproliferative thrombocytopenia. Transfus Med Rev 2015;29(1): 3–13.
5. Chang HY, Rodriguez V, Narboni G, et al. Causes of death in adults with acute leukemia. Medicine (Baltimore) 1976;55(3):259–68.
6. Leukocyte reduction and ultraviolet B irradiation of platelets to prevent alloimmunization and refractoriness to platelet transfusions. The Trial to Reduce Alloimmunization to Platelets Study Group. N Engl J Med 1997;337(26):1861–9.
7. Hod E, Schwartz J. Platelet transfusion refractoriness. Br J Haematol 2008; 142(3):348–60.
8. Brubaker DB, Marcus C, Holmes E. Intravascular and total body platelet equilibrium in healthy volunteers and in thrombocytopenic patients transfused with single donor platelets. Am J Hematol 1998;58(3):165–76.
9. O'Connell B, Lee EJ, Schiffer CA. The value of 10-minute posttransfusion platelet counts. Transfusion 1988;28(1):66–7.
10. Delaflor-Weiss E, Mintz PD. The evaluation and management of platelet refractoriness and alloimmunization. Transfus Med Rev 2000;14(2):180–96.
11. Schiffer CA, Anderson KC, Bennett CL, et al. Platelet transfusion for patients with cancer: clinical practice guidelines of the American Society of Clinical Oncology. J Clin Oncol 2001;19(5):1519–38.
12. Kopko PM, Warner P, Kresie L, et al. Methods for the selection of platelet products for alloimmune-refractory patients. Transfusion 2015;55(2):235–44.
13. Saito S, Ota S, Seshimo H, et al. Platelet transfusion refractoriness caused by a mismatch in HLA-C antigens. Transfusion 2002;42(3):302–8.
14. Claas FH, Smeenk RJ, Schmidt R, et al. Alloimmunization against the MHC antigens after platelet transfusions is due to contaminating leukocytes in the platelet suspension. Exp Hematol 1981;9(1):84–9.
15. Kickler T, Kennedy SD, Braine HG. Alloimmunization to platelet-specific antigens on glycoproteins IIb-IIIa and Ib/IX in multiply transfused thrombocytopenic patients. Transfusion 1990;30(7):622–5.
16. Godeau B, Fromont P, Seror T, et al. Platelet alloimmunization after multiple transfusions: a prospective study of 50 patients. Br J Haematol 1992;81(3):395–400.
17. McGrath K, Wolf M, Bishop J, et al. Transient platelet and HLA antibody formation in multitransfused patients with malignancy. Br J Haematol 1988;68(3):345–50.
18. Pappalardo PA, Secord AR, Quitevis P, et al. Platelet transfusion refractoriness associated with HPA-1a (Pl(A1)) alloantibody without coexistent HLA antibodies successfully treated with antigen-negative platelet transfusions. Transfusion 2001;41(8):984–7.

19. Dutcher JP, Schiffer CA, Aisner J, et al. Alloimmunization following platelet transfusion: the absence of a dose-response relationship. Blood 1981;57(3):395–8.
20. Schiffer CA, Lichtenfeld JL, Wiernik PH, et al. Antibody response in patients with acute nonlymphocytic leukemia. Cancer 1976;37(5):2177–82.
21. Dunstan RA, Simpson MB, Knowles RW, et al. The origin of ABH antigens on human platelets. Blood 1985;65(3):615–9.
22. Carr R, Hutton JL, Jenkins JA, et al. Transfusion of ABO-mismatched platelets leads to early platelet refractoriness. Br J Haematol 1990;75(3):408–13.
23. Bessos H, Atkinson A, McGill A, et al. Apheresis platelet concentrates: correlation of day one levels of in vitro quality markers with corresponding levels on days two to five of storage. Thromb Res 1996;84(5):367–72.
24. Slichter SJ, Davis K, Enright H, et al. Factors affecting posttransfusion platelet increments, platelet refractoriness, and platelet transfusion intervals in thrombocytopenic patients. Blood 2005;105(10):4106–14.
25. Legler TJ, Fischer I, Dittmann J, et al. Frequency and causes of refractoriness in multiply transfused patients. Ann Hematol 1997;74(4):185–9.
26. Klingemann HG, Self S, Banaji M, et al. Refractoriness to random donor platelet transfusions in patients with aplastic anaemia: a multivariate analysis of data from 264 cases. Br J Haematol 1987;66(1):115–21.
27. Doughty HA, Murphy MF, Metcalfe P, et al. Relative importance of immune and non-immune causes of platelet refractoriness. Vox Sang 1994;66(3):200–5.
28. Fontao-Wendel R, Silva LC, Saviolo CB, et al. Incidence of transfusion-induced platelet-reactive antibodies evaluated by specific assays for the detection of human leucocyte antigen and human platelet antigen antibodies. Vox Sang 2007; 93(3):241–9.
29. Yankee RA, Graff KS, Dowling R, et al. Selection of unrelated compatible platelet donors by lymphocyte HL-A matching. N Engl J Med 1973;288(15):760–4.
30. Duquesnoy RJ, Filip DJ, Rodey GE, et al. Successful transfusion of platelets "mismatched" for HLA antigens to alloimmunized thrombocytopenic patients. Am J Hematol 1977;2(3):219–26.
31. Moroff G, Garratty G, Heal JM, et al. Selection of platelets for refractory patients by HLA matching and prospective crossmatching. Transfusion 1992;32(7): 633–40.
32. Rioux-Masse B, Cohn C, Lindgren B, et al. Utilization of cross-matched or HLA-matched platelets for patients refractory to platelet transfusion. Transfusion 2014;54(12):3080–7.
33. Bolgiano DC, Larson EB, Slichter SJ. A model to determine required pool size for HLA-typed community donor apheresis programs. Transfusion 1989;29(4): 306–10.
34. Sacher RA, Kickler TS, Schiffer CA, et al. Management of patients refractory to platelet transfusion. Arch Pathol Lab Med 2003;127(4):409–14.
35. Rebulla P, Morelati F, Revelli N, et al. Outcomes of an automated procedure for the selection of effective platelets for patients refractory to random donors based on cross-matching locally available platelet products. Br J Haematol 2004;125(1): 83–9.
36. Vassallo RR, Fung M, Rebulla P, et al. Utility of cross-matched platelet transfusions in patients with hypoproliferative thrombocytopenia: a systematic review. Transfusion 2014;54(4):1180–91.
37. Myers TJ, Kim BK, Steiner M, et al. Selection of donor platelets for alloimmunized patients using a platelet-associated IgG assay. Blood 1981;58(3):444–50.

38. Petz LD, Garratty G, Calhoun L, et al. Selecting donors of platelets for refractory patients on the basis of HLA antibody specificity. Transfusion 2000;40(12): 1446–56.

39. Dunbar NM, Ornstein DL, Dumont LJ. ABO incompatible platelets: risks versus benefit. Curr Opin Hematol 2012;19(6):475–9.

40. Aster RH, Bougie DW. Drug-induced immune thrombocytopenia. N Engl J Med 2007;357(6):580–7.

41. Tinmouth AT, Semple E, Shehata N, et al. Platelet immunopathology and therapy: a Canadian Blood Services Research and Development Symposium. Transfus Med Rev 2006;20(4):294–314.

42. Kam T, Alexander M. Drug-induced immune thrombocytopenia. J Pharm Pract 2014;27(5):430–9.

43. Kalmadi S, Tiu R, Lowe C, et al. Epsilon aminocaproic acid reduces transfusion requirements in patients with thrombocytopenic hemorrhage. Cancer 2006; 107(1):136–40.

44. Ben-Bassat I, Douer D, Ramot B. Tranexamic acid therapy in acute myeloid leukemia: possible reduction of platelet transfusions. Eur J Haematol 1990;45(2): 86–9.

45. Avvisati G, ten Cate JW, Buller HR, et al. Tranexamic acid for control of haemorrhage in acute promyelocytic leukaemia. Lancet 1989;2(8655):122–4.

46. Antun AG, Gleason S, Arellano M, et al. Epsilon aminocaproic acid prevents bleeding in severely thrombocytopenic patients with hematological malignancies. Cancer 2013;119(21):3784–7.

47. Ratko TA, Burnett DA, Foulke GE, et al. Recommendations for off-label use of intravenously administered immunoglobulin preparations. University Hospital Consortium Expert Panel for Off-Label Use of Polyvalent Intravenously Administered Immunoglobulin Preparations. JAMA 1995;273(23):1865–70.

48. Kickler T. Pretransfusion testing for platelet transfusions. Transfusion 2000;40(12): 1425–6.

49. Schiffer CA, Hogge DE, Aisner J, et al. High-dose intravenous gammaglobulin in alloimmunized platelet transfusion recipients. Blood 1984;64(4):937–40.

50. Hogge DE, Dutcher JP, Aisner J, et al. The ineffectiveness of random donor platelet transfusion in splenectomized, alloimmunized recipients. Blood 1984; 64(1):253–6.

51. Heddle NM, Klama L, Kelton JG, et al. The use of anti-D to improve post-transfusion platelet response: a randomized trial. Br J Haematol 1995;89(1): 163–8.

52. Christie DJ, Howe RB, Lennon SS, et al. Treatment of refractoriness to platelet transfusion by protein A column therapy. Transfusion 1993;33(3):234–42.

53. Nagasawa T, Kim BK, Baldini MG. Temporary suppression of circulating antiplatelet alloantibodies by the massive infusion of fresh, stored, or lyophilized platelets. Transfusion 1978;18(4):429–35.

54. Narvios A, Reddy V, Martinez F, et al. Slow infusion of platelets: a possible alternative in the management of refractory thrombocytopenic patients. Am J Hematol 2005;79(1):80.

55. Heuer L, Blumenberg D. Management of bleeding in a multi-transfused patient with positive HLA class I alloantibodies and thrombocytopenia associated with platelet dysfunction refractory to transfusion of cross-matched platelets. Blood Coagul Fibrinolysis 2005;16(4):287–90.

56. Vidarsson B, Onundarson PT. Recombinant factor VIIa for bleeding in refractory thrombocytopenia. Thromb Haemost 2000;83(4):634–5.

Management of Thrombotic Microangiopathic Hemolytic Anemias with Therapeutic Plasma Exchange
When It Works and When It Does Not

Tahir Mehmood, MD[a], Michelle Taylor, MD[b],
Jeffrey L. Winters, MD[c],*

KEYWORDS

- Plasma exchange • Plasmapheresis • Thrombotic microangiopathy
- Thrombotic thrombocytopenic purpura • Hemolytic uremic syndrome • Apheresis

KEY POINTS

- Thrombotic microangiopathies (TMA) are inherited and acquired disorders characterized by microangiopathic hemolytic anemia, thrombocytopenia, and organ damage resulting from microvasculature occlusion.
- Randomized controlled trials involving plasma exchange (TPE) exist only for thrombotic thrombocytopenic purpura (TTP) with evidence supporting use in other TMA consisting of low- to very low-quality evidence.
- The American Society for Apheresis considers TPE ineffective for the treatment of Shiga toxin–mediated TMA, selected complement-mediated TMA, and selected drug-associated TMA.
- The usual course of TPE applied to TTP is usually applied to the other TMA.
- The usual replacement fluid used in TMA is plasma, with the exception of *Streptococcus pneumoniae*-associated hemolytic uremic syndrome, where albumin is the suggested replacement fluid.

The authors have no commercial or financial conflicts of interest or funding sources related to this article or the topics of thrombotic microangiopathies and their treatment.

[a] Division of Hospital Internal Medicine, Department of Internal Medicine, Mayo Clinic, 200 First Street Southwest, Rochester, MN 55905, USA; [b] Transfuse Solutions, Inc, 413 9th Avenue Northwest, Byron, MN 55920, USA; [c] Division of Transfusion Medicine, Department of Laboratory Medicine and Pathology, Mayo Clinic, 200 First Street Southwest, Rochester, MN 55905, USA
* Corresponding author.
E-mail address: winters.jeffrey@mayo.edu

INTRODUCTION

Thrombotic microangiopathies (TMA) are a heterogeneous group of disorders, some inherited and some acquired, that share common clinical features. These features are microangiopathic hemolytic anemia (MAHA) (**Box 1**), thrombocytopenia, and organ damage due to microvasculature endothelial damage.[1] Although several disorders are considered to be TMA, this review is limited to those for which the use of plasma exchange (TPE) has been described in the medical literature. The disorders discussed are briefly described in **Table 1**. Of note, in addition to the traditional names used, **Table 1** also provides alternate names, where available, in parentheses as recommended by George and Nester.[1] These suggested alternate names are intended to provide clarity when discussing these disorders by describing the cause of the TMA.[1]

TPE is a medical procedure whereby plasma is removed and replaced with a colloid or a combination of a colloid and crystalloid replacement fluid.[2] The potential mechanisms of actions of TPE are numerous and vary according to the disease entity being considered.[3] In the case of the TMA, possible mechanisms of action include the removal of pathologic antibodies, the removal of abnormal plasma proteins, and the replacement of absent or abnormal plasma proteins.[3] The American Society for Apheresis (ASFA) provides guidance on the use of TPE in the treatment of many, but not all, of the TMA.[2] The role of apheresis therapy in the treatment of a disorder is defined by the ASFA category, with the ASFA recommendation grade providing an indication of the strength of the recommendation to perform the procedure and the quality of the published evidence supporting the treatment. These ASFA categories and the ASFA recommendation grade are defined in **Box 2** and **Table 2**, respectively, and given for each disorder, where available, in **Table 1**. Key considerations in using TPE to treat any disorder are listed in **Box 3** and are again described for many of the TMA in the ASFA guidelines. This information is provided in the sections discussing the various TMA.

THROMBOTIC THROMBOCYTOPENIC PURPURA (ADAMTS13 DEFICIENCY-MEDIATED THROMBOTIC MICROANGIOPATHIES)

Thrombotic thrombocytopenic purpura (TTP) is a rare disorder that carries a high risk of mortality if prompt treatment is not initiated. ADAMTS13 (a disintegrin and metalloproteinase with a thrombospondin type 1 motif, member 13) is a proteolytic enzyme that cleaves ultra-large von Willebrand factor multimers (UvWF) into smaller monomers. Congenital absence of ADAMTS13 or presence of an inhibitor leading to decreased activity level has been established as the underlying pathophysiology of TTP. UvWF circulate in the plasma and bind platelets leading to microthrombi in small blood vessels, resulting in clinical manifestations of TTP including MAHA,

---

Box 1
Features of microangiopathic hemolytic anemia

- Anemia
- Schistocytes
- Decreased haptoglobin
- Elevated LDH

thrombocytopenia, renal failure, fever, and neurologic changes. When a patient presents with anemia and thrombocytopenia, an urgent evaluation is warranted to rule out TTP. Peripheral smear suggestive of MAHA and the presence of thrombocytopenia are sufficient indicators to initiate TPE according to current recommendations.[2,4] Rock and colleagues[5] demonstrated that TPE was superior to plasma infusion in TTP patients in a randomized trial. In cases whereby TPE is not available, plasma infusion should be used because equivalence has been demonstrated when large volumes of plasma are infused.[6] However, these volumes carry a high risk of volume overload, particularly if the patient has developed renal failure from their TTP.[6] ADAMTS13 level and inhibitor level are checked on the pre-TPE blood sample, because levels have important prognostic and diagnostic implications. Patients with undetectable ADAMTS13 levels at the initiation of TPE have a higher survival rate (82%) when compared with patients with detectable levels (46%),[7] and patients with ADAMTS13 activity less than 10% have a higher risk of relapse.[8] During TPE, ADAMTS13 is replaced, whereas inhibitory antibodies and UvWF are removed.[4]

The usual treatment course, as recommended by ASFA, as well as criteria for discontinuing TPE is given in **Box 4**. Of note, the disappearance of schistocytes is not a criterion for discontinuation of TPE because their presence or absence is not correlated with relapse.[9] In addition, there is also no evidence supporting the superiority of abruptly discontinuing TPE versus weaning TPE once the criteria outlined in **Box 4** have been achieved.[10] TPE replacement fluid used must contain ADAMTS13 and have included fresh frozen plasma (FFP), thawed plasma, methylene blue–photoactivated plasma,[11] solvent detergent-treated plasma,[12] and plasma, cryoprecipitate reduced.[13] del Rio-Garma and colleagues,[11] however, found methylene blue–photoactivated plasma inferior to FFP. Theoretically, solvent detergent-treated plasma and plasma, cryoprecipitate reduced, because of reduced vWF, should offer benefits over FFP. A randomized trial, however, failed to demonstrate a benefit of plasma, cryoprecipitate reduced in patients with TTP at initial presentation.[13]

If there is no response to TPE after 7 days, the addition of high-dose steroids, addition of rituximab, or twice daily TPE can be considered.[14,15] In refractory patients, the use of plasma, cryoprecipitate reduced as a replacement fluid has demonstrated increased response.[16]

INFECTION-ASSOCIATED THROMBOTIC THROMBOCYTOPENIC PURPURA
Human immunodeficiency virus-associated Thrombotic Thrombocytopenic Purpura

TTP occurs rarely in human immunodeficiency virus (HIV) patients. In most of these patients, ADAMTS13 level is low, and inhibitory antibodies are detected.[17] A retrospective study looking at HIV and TMA noted up to 33% of patients presented with TTP as their initial HIV presentation.[18] HIV patients with poor compliance to highly active antiretroviral therapy (HAART) and low CD4 counts are at risk for TTP.[18] Initiation of TPE and HAART therapy concurrently results in significant reduction in TTP mortality.[18] The course of TPE therapy outlined in **Box 4** is usually initiated, with HAART medications administered after TPE.[18] When TPE is not available or there is a delay in initiating TPE, plasma transfusion along with steroids should be considered.[18] Although not statistically significant, high viral load was associated with greater number of TPE necessary for remission.[18] After discontinuation of TPE, HAART therapy should be continued to reduce TTP recurrence.[18] Currently, HIV-associated TTP is not categorized by ASFA.[2]

Table 1
Thrombotic microangiopathies treated with plasma exchange

Disorder[a]	Pathophysiology	Patient Population	Signs and Symptoms	ASFA Category[2]	ASFA Recommendation Grade[2]
TTP (ADAMTS13 deficiency-mediated TMA)	Deficiency of ADAMTS13 activity due to either congenital deficiency or development of inhibitory autoantibodies	Adults or children	MAHA, thrombocytopenia, fever, neurologic symptoms, renal dysfunction	I	1A
Shiga toxin–associated HUS or typical HUS or diarrhea-associated HUS (ST-TMA)	Direct endothelial damage due to toxic effects of Shiga toxin	Predominantly a disease of children <5 y of age	MAHA, thrombocytopenia, renal dysfunction, bloody diarrhea	IV	1C
pHUS	Endothelial damage due to crypt antigen exposure or inhibition of Factor H due to protein damage leading to unregulated complement activation	A disease of children <2 y of age associated predominantly with S pneumoniae pneumonia	MAHA, thrombocytopenia, and acute kidney injury	III	2C
aHUS (complement-mediated TMA)	Endothelial damage due to unregulated complement activation	Adults or children	MAHA, thrombocytopenia, and acute kidney injury	Complement gene Mutations—II Membrane cofactor mutations—IV Factor H autoantibodies—I	Complement gene Mutations—2C Membrane cofactor mutations—1C Factor H autoantibodies—2C

HSCT-TMA	Endothelial damage due to infection, chemotherapy, radiation therapy, and/or GVHD	Adults or children	MAHA, thrombocytopenia, renal failure, and neurologic symptoms	III	2C
Renal transplant-associated TMA	Endothelial damage due to calcineurin inhibitors and possibly other transplant-related factors	Renal transplant patients	MAHA, thrombocytopenia, and worsening or delayed graft function	NC	NC
Drug-associated TMA (drug-mediated TMA immune reaction or drug-mediated TMA toxic dose-related reaction)	See **Table 3**	Adults or children	MAHA, thrombocytopenia, and renal failure	See **Table 3**	See **Table 3**
Malignancy-associated TMA	Coagulation cascade activation due to tumor tissue factor expression	Adults with cancer, predominantly adenocarcinomas	MAHA, thrombocytopenia, bone pain, respiratory symptoms, anorexia, and weight loss	NC	NC

Abbreviations: ADAMTS13, a disintegrin and metalloproteinase with a thrombospondin type 1 motif, member 13; ASFA, American Society for Apheresis; GVHD, graft-versus-host disease; NC, not categorized.

[a] Names in parentheses suggested by George and Nester[1] for clarity.

Data from George JN, Nester CM. Syndromes of thrombotic microangiopathy. N Engl J Med 2014;371:654–66; and Schwartz J, Winters JL, Padmanabhan A, et al. Guidelines on the use of therapeutic apheresis in clinical practice—evidence-based approach from the apheresis applications committee of the American Society for Apheresis. The sixth special issue. J Clin Apher 2013;28:145–284.

Box 2
American Society for Apheresis recommendation grade definitions

Strong recommendation: 1

Weak recommendation: 2

High-quality evidence (eg, randomized, double-blinded, controlled trials): A
Moderate-quality evidence (eg, controlled trials): B
Low- or very low-quality evidence (eg, case series or reports, expert opinion): C

From Schwartz J, Winters JL, Padmanabhan A, et al. Guidelines on the use of therapeutic apheresis in clinical practice—evidence-based approach from the apheresis applications committee of the American Society for Apheresis. The sixth special issue. J Clin Apher 2013;28:147,148; with permission.

INFECTION-ASSOCIATED HEMOLYTIC UREMIC SYNDROME
Typical Hemolytic Uremic Syndrome, Diarrhea-associated Hemolytic Uremic Syndrome, or Shiga Toxin–associated Hemolytic Uremic Syndrome (Shiga Toxin–mediated Thrombotic Microangiopathies)

Shiga toxin–producing *Escherichia coli* is the most common type of infection-associated hemolytic uremic syndrome (HUS) with other causative organisms, including *Shigella dysenteriae* and *Yersinia* species.[19] Unlike TTP, ADAMTS13 does not appear to have a role in Shiga toxin–mediated TMA (ST-TMA) with the MAHA resulting from direct endothelial injury from the toxin.[19] This disorder is predominantly a pediatric disorder and is most commonly seen in those less than 5 years of age.[19]

Given the lack of antibodies or abnormal plasma proteins, the role of TPE in this disorder is not clear. An observational study of 5 patients involved in a European ST-TMA outbreak found early improvement in patients undergoing TPE.[20] A larger retrospective analysis of German ST-TMA registry examining the outcomes among a much larger cohort of patients receiving supportive care, TPE, or TPE and eculizumab, found no differences in outcomes among the different interventions.[21] A case controlled study of this same German outbreak also evaluated these treatment strategies and found no benefits of steroids, TPE, or eculizumab.[22]

There is a lack of efficacy data on the utility of TPE in ST-TMA.[2] It has been suggested by some investigators that patients with severe neurologic symptoms or risk of death at presentation should be started on TPE.[23] This suggestion represents

---

Table 2
American Society for Apheresis category definitions

Category	Definition
I	Accepted first-line therapy, stand-alone or as an adjunct to other therapies
II	Second-line therapy, stand-alone or as an adjunct to other therapies
III	Optimum role of apheresis is uncertain, decision-making should be individualized based on each patient's clinical situation
IV	Apheresis therapy ineffective or harmful

From Schwartz J, Winters JL, Padmanabhan A, et al. Guidelines on the use of therapeutic apheresis in clinical practice—evidence-based approach from the apheresis applications committee of the American Society for Apheresis. The sixth special issue. J Clin Apher 2013;28:147; with permission.

Box 3
Key considerations in treating thrombotic microangiopathies with plasma exchange

- Volume of plasma exchanged
- Fluid used to replace the removed plasma
- Frequency of treatment
- Length of treatment

---

opinion opposed to evidence-based practice, however. ASFA categorizes ST-TMA as category IV indication, indicating the treatment is ineffective or harmful; this appears to be especially true in pediatric patients whereby the use of TPE is associated with increased complications related to the procedure.[2] Early use of the antibiotics has been suggested to be beneficial in improving the outcomes in ST-HUS patients.[22,23]

Streptococcus pneumoniae–associated hemolytic uremic syndrome

Acute hemolytic anemia, thrombocytopenia, and renal injury in the setting of *Streptococcus pneumoniae* infection suggest *S pneumonia*–associated HUS (pHUS).[2,24] Since its first description in 1971, pHUS has been observed in pediatric patients, predominantly less than 2 years of age, suffering from *S pneumoniae* pneumonia or meningitis. The former accounts for most cases.[24] The pathophysiology of the disorder is uncertain, but it is thought that neuraminidase produced by *S pneumoniae* cleaves the sialic acid residues from the surface of red blood cells (RBCs), platelets, and endothelial cells exposing Thomsen-Friedenreich (TF) antigen. Naturally occurring immunoglobulin M antibody against the TF antigen causes RBC agglutination and endothelial injury.[24] More recently, it has been suggested that the neuraminidase may remove sialic acid residues from Factor H binding sites such that it cannot interact with C3 convertase or through direct inhibition of Factor H.[24] In either case, the result would be unregulated complement activation.[24]

Supportive care along with the avoidance of plasma and use of washed cellular blood products, when needed, is the usual course of therapy.[24,25] Washing is performed to remove residual plasma, which would contain antibodies to the TF antigen. Some patients may present with severe sepsis and multiorgan failure, in which

---

Box 4
American Society for Apheresis recommendations for plasma exchange in thrombotic microangiopathies

- Frequency of TPE: daily
- Plasma volume replaced: 1 to 1.5
- Replacement fluid: plasma[a]

- Discontinuation: resolution of neurologic symptoms (if applicable), platelet count greater than 150×10^9/L, and LDH near normal for 2 to 3 consecutive days.

[a] Except pHUS whereby albumin is recommended.
From Schwartz J, Winters JL, Padmanabhan A, et al. Guidelines on the use of therapeutic apheresis in clinical practice—evidence-based approach from the apheresis applications committee of the American Society for Apheresis. The sixth special issue. J Clin Apher 2013;28:232; with permission.

case TPE using albumin as a replacement has been suggested.[25] Some reports have suggested using "low titer anti-TF plasma,"[26] although "low titer" is not defined. It is postulated that TPE could remove the circulating anti-TF and neuraminidase.[24,25] Evidence, however, is limited to case series and case reports without an obvious difference noted in patient outcomes with TPE versus supportive care.[25] Current ASFA recommendations are provided in **Box 4**.

Atypical Hemolytic Uremic Syndrome (Complement Regulatory Pathway-associated Hemolytic Uremic Syndrome or Complement-mediated Thrombotic Microangiopathies)

Atypical HUS (aHUS) is a life-threatening TMA with acute renal failure occurring in the absence of the infectious agents mentioned previously. The underlying pathophysiology involves the dysregulation of the alternative complement pathway, through either mutations resulting in loss of function in complement regulatory proteins (eg, complement factor H [CFH], complement factor I), mutations resulting in gain in function in complement pathway components (eg, complement factor B and C3), or the presence of inhibitory autoantibodies to regulatory proteins (eg, anti-CFH).[27,28] The result is excessive complement activation on the microvasculature surface leading to TMA.[27,28] In the past, up to 73% of the patients developed end-stage renal failure within 5 years following the diagnosis and, depending on the mutations involved, up to 100% develop recurrence in transplanted kidneys.[27]

The goal of therapy in aHUS is to prevent the worsening of renal function and need for renal transplantation. Addition of normal complement proteins and removal of their dysfunctional counterparts along with removal of autoantibodies and inflammatory cytokines is achieved by TPE using plasma as the replacement fluid.[27,28] Long-term maintenance TPE has been suggested as renal protective compared with short-term TPE followed by plasma infusion, but with the recent availability of eculizumab as an inhibitor of the complement pathway, the use of this medication has become the preferred method for controlling aHUS and preventing end-stage renal disease.[27,28]

Currently TPE is the first-line therapy for aHUS in patients with evidence of acute exacerbation.[2,28] Because patients may present with TTP-like features, TPE is initiated promptly and evaluation of ADAMTS13 activity and inhibitor levels along with tests of the complement cascade are obtained.[28] Patients are monitored closely for the efficacy of TPE. No response to TPE and greater than 10% ADAMTS13 activity suggest aHUS, and eculizumab should be considered for further acute treatment.[28] As evidence suggests that a more rapid initiation of eculizumab is associated with better renal outcomes, it should be initiated as soon as the diagnosis is confirmed.[28] The required duration of eculizumab therapy is currently unknown but exacerbations of aHUS occur, and therefore, life-long treatment may be required. Patient characteristics that determine this need to be further elucidated.[28] ASFA recommends TPE in some but not all complement-mediated TMA (see **Table 1**), depending on the mutation that is present. For example, mutations in membrane cofactor protein, a membrane-bound complement regulatory protein, have good outcomes regardless of the use of TPE, and as a membrane-bound protein, would not be affected by TPE. As a result, this is a category IV indication for TPE, and apheresis is ineffective or harmful.[2]

HEMATOPOIETIC STEM CELL TRANSPLANT-ASSOCIATED THROMBOTIC MICROANGIOPATHIES

Hematopoietic stem cell transplant–associated thrombotic microangiopathy (HSCT-TMA) presents in transplant patients as thrombocytopenia, MAHA, renal dysfunction, and neurologic symptoms.[29] Existing literature on HSCT-TMA is inconsistent with regard to many aspects of the condition, such as incidence, pathogenesis, and optimal therapeutic measures, because of the use of varied diagnostic criteria.[30] Currently, 2 sets of diagnostic criteria for HSCT-TMA are widely used. The International Working Group criteria require greater than 4% schistocytes on peripheral smear, de novo prolonged or progressive thrombocytopenia, sudden and persistent increase in lactate dehydrogenase (LDH) concentration, decrease in hemoglobin concentration or increased transfusion requirement, and decrease in serum haptoglobin.[31] The Blood and Marrow Transplant Clinical Trials Network Toxicity Committee criteria include RBC fragmentation and at least 2 schistocytes per high-power-field on peripheral smear, increased LDH, concurrent unexplained renal and/or neurologic dysfunction, and negative direct and indirect antiglobulin tests.[32] In addition, patients with HSCT-TMA have greater than 5% ADAMTS13 activity and normal vWF multimeric patterns.[30]

The final common pathway for HSCT-TMA, like many other TMA, is endothelial injury.[33] A variety of possible causes of injury exist in the transplant setting and are listed in **Box 5**. These causes may be further affected by other patient factors including circulating cytokines, circulating endothelial cells, abnormalities in the coagulation cascade, and mutations in complement regulatory pathways, such as seen with aHUS.[33] Poor prognostic indicators in HSCT-TMA are listed in **Box 6**.

The effectiveness of TPE in treatment of HSCT-TMA is uncertain.[33] Ho and colleagues[32] found a median response rate to TPE of 36.5% (range 0%–80%) with a mortality of 80% in reports published between 1991 and 2003. Laskin and colleagues[33] found a response rate of 27% to 80% in series published from 2003 to 2011. None of these reports represented controlled trials, and the only prospective study, which involved TPE and discontinuation of cyclosporine, demonstrated a response rate of 64%.[33] Most recommendations for therapy involve treatment and/ or elimination of potential causes of endothelial damage as listed in **Box 5**.[29,30,33] Evidence does exist that TPE may be effective in HSCT-TMA when acute graft-versus-host disease is absent.[29] However, given that TPE is also associated with several complications, benefits may not outweigh risks.[30,33] Because of the uncertainty of the efficacy of TPE, ASFA has indicated that the optimal role of TPE is uncertain (category III).[2]

RENAL TRANSPLANT-ASSOCIATED THROMBOTIC MICROANGIOPATHIES

TMA occurs in 3% to 14% of renal transplant patients receiving calcineurin immunosuppression with a presentation that includes MAHA, thrombocytopenia, and

---

Box 5
Potential causes of endothelial damage in hematopoietic stem cell transplant-associated thrombotic microangiopathies

- Infection

- Chemotherapy

- Radiation therapy

- Graft-versus-host disease

Data from Laskin BL, Goebel J, Davies SM, et al. Small vessel, big trouble in the kidneys and beyond: hematopoietic stem cell transplantation-associated thrombotic microangiopathy. Blood 2011;118:1452–62.

Box 6
Poor prognostic indicators in hematopoietic stem cell transplant-associated thrombotic microangiopathies

- Age greater than 18 years
- Unrelated or haploidentical graft source
- Five or more schistocytes per high-power-field on peripheral smear
- Thrombotic microangiopathy in the absence of sirolimus exposure
- Nephropathy

From Choi CM, Schmaier AH, Snell MR, et al. Thrombotic microangiopathy in haematopoietic stem cell transplantation diagnosis and treatment. Drugs 2009;69:188; with permission.

worsening or delayed graft function.[34] Risk factors for the development of renal transplant-associated TMA are provided in **Box 7**. Renal transplant-associated TMA may present localized to the allograft or as a systemic disorder similar to aHUS.[34] In either setting, the diagnosis is confirmed by a combination of renal biopsy findings and laboratory testing.[34] Reynolds and colleagues[35] found peak incidence of the development of renal transplant-associated TMA occurred 3 to 6 months after transplant, although risk continued beyond this time frame. Cyclosporine and tacrolimus immunosuppression have been associated with renal transplant-associated TMA with the major therapeutic intervention being reduction or temporary withdrawal of these medications.[34,36] Of note, reintroduction of calcineurin inhibitors was not associated with recurrence of the disorder.[36] In the study of Schwimmer and colleagues,[34] patients with systemic symptoms were more likely to undergo TPE, but there was no difference in graft loss in those who had TPE and those who did not, regardless of the presence or absence of systemic symptoms. They were not able to draw any conclusions about the benefit of TPE. Caires and colleagues[36] found TPE resulted in durable remission in 80% of their renal transplant-associated TMA patients, but graft survival remained poor regardless of the treatment used. ASFA has not provided recommendations on the use of TPE in renal transplant-associated TMA.[2]

MALIGNANCY-ASSOCIATED THROMBOTIC MICROANGIOPATHIES

In patients with malignancy, the presence of MAHA with thrombocytopenia has been well documented.[37] The diagnostic criteria for malignancy-associated TMA are provided in **Box 8**. In the study by Elliot and colleagues,[37] the median hemoglobin was

Box 7
Risk factors for renal transplant-associated thrombotic microangiopathies

- Female recipient
- Sirolimus therapy
- Younger recipient age
- Older donor age

Data from Reynolds JC, Agodoa LY, Yuan CM, et al. Thrombotic microangiopathy after renal transplantation in the United States. Am J Kidney Dis 2003;42:1058–68.

> **Box 8**
> **Diagnostic criteria for malignancy-associated thrombotic microangiopathies**
>
> • Diagnosis of cancer
>
> • Direct antiglobulin negative hemolytic anemia with schistocytes and thrombocytopenia
>
> • Decreased serum haptoglobin
>
> • Indirect hyperbilirubinemia
>
> *Data from* Elliott MA, Letendre L, Gastineau DA, et al. Cancer-associated microangiopathic he-
> molytic anemia with thrombocytopenia: an important diagnostic consideration. Eur J Haema-
> tol 2010;85:43–50; and Lechner K, Obermeier HL. Cancer-related microangiopathic hemolytic
> anemia clinical and laboratory features in 168 reported cases. Medicine 2012;91:195–205.

6.9 g/dL and the median platelet count was 18×10^9/L; all patients had elevated
D-dimer levels with the absence of other features of disseminated intravascular coagulation (DIC), and the median serum creatinine was 1.2 mg/dL. ADAMTS13 activity is
greater than 10% or normal in malignancy-associated TMA.[37–39] In addition to these
laboratory findings, patients with malignancy-associated TMA may present with
higher frequencies of bone pain, respiratory symptoms, anorexia, and weight loss
compared with patients with TTP.[37,39,40] Compared with patients with idiopathic
TMA, patients with malignancy-associated TMA were older and had a longer history
of symptoms preceding diagnosis.[39]

The pathogenesis of malignancy-associated TMA is unclear, but may be related to
antineoplastic drugs used to treat the malignancy or to the cancer itself through the
activation of the coagulation cascade by expression of tissue factor on widespread tumor.[40] Favre and colleagues[41] described 2 malignancy-associated TMA patients in
whom underlying CFH mutations, identical to those reported in aHUS, were present,
suggesting that such mutations in complement cascade regulation may be involved.
The most common cancers associated with malignancy-associated TMA are adeno-
carcinomas of the stomach, breast, prostate, and lung as well as cancers of unknown
primary.[42]

Prognosis of malignancy-associated TMA is poor. TPE has shown no benefit and
may actually be more harmful to the patient because it may delay the initiation of
cancer-specific chemotherapy.[37,39,40] ASFA has not provided recommendations for
the use of TPE in malignancy-associated TMA.[2]

DRUG-ASSOCIATED THROMBOTIC MICROANGIOPATHIES (DRUG-MEDIATED THROMBOTIC MICROANGIOPATHIES IMMUNE REACTION OR DRUG-MEDIATED THROMBOTIC MICROANGIOPATHIES TOXIC DOSE-RELATED REACTION)

A wide variety of drugs have been implicated in the development of TMA. In a recent
systemic review, a total of 78 different medications had been reported to be associated with TMA.[43] However, a definitive causal association was only present in
22 (28%) of the drugs based on the criteria used by the investigators in their review.[43]
As with other TMA syndromes, the presentation is usually one of MAHA, thrombocytopenia, and renal failure. The mechanisms behind the development of TMA varies
depending on the drug and includes direct injury to endothelium, frequently in a
dose-dependent manner, immune-mediated reactions with the development of
drug-dependent antibodies, and, in at least one instance, the development of inhibitory antibodies to ADAMTS13 similar to that seen in TTP.[43–45] Those medications
for which definitive evidence for an association with drug-mediated TMA are listed
in **Box 9**.[43,44]

Box 9
Drugs with definitive causal association with drug-associated thrombotic microangiopathies

- Drugs identified in a systemic review[43]
  - Cyclosporine
  - Quinine
  - Tacrolimus
- Drugs identified based on registry review using stringent criteria[44]
  - Gemcitabine
  - Pentostatin
  - Quinine
- Drugs identified based on laboratory testing with the presence of antidrug antibodies[44]
  - Oxaliplatin
  - Quinine
  - Vancomycin

Data from Al-Nouri ZL, Reese JA, Terrell DR, et al. Drug-induced thrombotic microangiopathy: a systemic review of published reports. Blood 2015;125:616–8; and Reese JA, Bougie DW, Curtis BR, et al. Drug-induced thrombotic microangiopathy: experience of the Oklahoma Registry and the BloodCenter of Wisconsin. Am J Hematol 2015;90:406–10.

The primary treatment of drug-associated TMA is discontinuation of the implicated medication. In the case of the calcineurin inhibitors, such as cyclosporine and tacrolimus, where it may not be possible to discontinue the drug, dose reduction and switching to another calcineurin inhibitor have also been effective.[45] In addition, there have been reports of successfully restarting cyclosporine following resolution of the

---

Table 3
Drugs reported to cause drug-associated thrombotic microangiopathies, pathophysiology, and American Society for Apheresis classification

Drug	Pathophysiology	ASFA Category	ASFA Recommendation Grade
Thienopyridines			
Ticlopidine	Development of ADAMTS13 autoantibodies	I	2B
Clopidogrel	Direct endothelial damage	III	1B
Calcineurin inhibitors			
Cyclosporine	Direct endothelial damage	III	2C
Tacrolimus	Direct endothelial damage	III	2C
Nucleoside analogues			
Gemcitabine	Direct endothelial damage	IV	2C
Mitomycin-C	Direct endothelial damage	NC	NC
Antiangiogenic factors			
Bevacizumab	Injury to renal podocytes	NC	NC
Sunitinib	Injury to renal podocytes	NC	NC
VEGF trap	Injury to renal podocytes	NC	NC
Other			
Quinine	Development of drug dependent antibodies	IV	2C

Abbreviations: NC, not classified; VEGF, vascular endothelial growth factor.
Data from Refs.[2,43,45]

TMA.[45] The role of TPE in the drug-associated TMA is unclear. In the case of ticlopidine, the presence of decreased ADAMTS13 activity and inhibitors as well as survival of 87% of patients when treated with TPE suggests efficacy. The absence of decreased ADAMTS13 activity and inhibitors and a 50% response rate being reported with TPE in the case of clopidogrel suggest that TPE may not be effective.[45] For cyclosporine and tacrolimus, the mechanism of direct endothelial injury suggests that TPE would not be effective; however, ASFA has categorized its role as uncertain (**Table 3**). Similarly, the direct endothelial injury caused by gemcitabine and mitomycin-C suggests a lack of efficacy of TPE. In one study, 18% of patients with gemcitabine-induced TMA treated with TPE recovered compared with 56% who did not receive TPE.[45] For mitomycin-C, 70% of patients treated with TPE either had no response or did worse.[45] For the antiangiogenic factors, the published evidence is limited, and therefore, the role of TPE is unclear. ASFA recommendations for these medications are provided in **Table 3**. When TPE is performed, the course of therapy is that as outlined in **Box 4**.

SUMMARY

Thrombotic microangiopathy represents a set of findings that results from a heterogeneous group of inherited and acquired disorders. Of the various causes, TTP is the only TMA whereby TPE has been evaluated using randomized controlled trials. For all of the remaining disorders, TPE has been applied because of the response of TTP. For disorders such as pHUS, HSCT-TMA, and renal transplant-associated TMA, the optimum role of TPE is uncertain. For ST-TMA and the malignancy-associated TMA, there appears to be no role for TPE. For the drug-associated TMA and complement-mediated TMA, the role of TPE varies depending on the drug involved and the complement pathway abnormality present. Further study is needed to definitively ascertain the role of TPE in treating these disorders.

REFERENCES

1. George JN, Nester CM. Syndromes of thrombotic microangiopathy. N Engl J Med 2014;371:654–66.
2. Schwartz J, Winters JL, Padmanabhan A, et al. Guidelines on the use of therapeutic apheresis in clinical practice—evidence-based approach from the Apheresis Applications Committee of the American Society for Apheresis. The sixth special issue. J Clin Apher 2013;28:145–284.
3. Reeves HM, Winters JL. The mechanisms of action of plasma exchange. Br J Haematol 2014;164:342–51.
4. Sarode R, Bandarenko N, Brecher ME, et al. Thrombotic thrombocytopenic purpura: 2012 American Society for Apheresis (ASFA) consensus conference on classification, diagnosis, management, and future research. J Clin Apher 2014;29:148–67.
5. Rock GA, Shumak KH, Buskard NA, et al. Comparison of plasma exchange with plasma infusion in the treatment of thrombotic thrombocytopenic purpura. The Canadian Apheresis Study Group. N Engl J Med 1991;325:393–7.
6. Coppo P, Bussel A, Charrier S, et al. High-dose plasma infusion versus plasma exchange as early treatment of thrombotic thrombocytopenic purpura/hemolytic-uremic syndrome. Medicine 2003;82:27–38.
7. Zheng XL, Kaufman RM, Goodnough LT, et al. Effect of plasma exchange on plasma ADAMTS13 metalloprotease activity, inhibitor level and clinical outcome

in patients with idiopathic and nonidiopathic thrombotic thrombocytopenic purpura. Blood 2004;103:4043–9.

8. Kremer Hovinga JA, Vesely SK, Terrell DR, et al. Survival and relapse in patients with thrombotic thrombocytopenic purpura. Blood 2010;115:1500–11.

9. Egan JA, Hay SN, Brecher ME. Frequency and significance of schistocytes in TTP/HUS patients at the discontinuation of plasma exchange therapy. J Clin Apher 2004;19:165–7.

10. Bandarenko N, Brecher ME. US TTP Apheresis Study Group. United States Thrombotic Thrombocytopenic Purpura Apheresis Study Group (US TTP ASG): multicenter survey and retrospective analysis of current efficacy of therapeutic plasma exchange. J Clin Apher 1998;13:133–41.

11. del Rio-Garma J, Alvarez-Larran A, Muncunill J, et al. Methylene blue-photoactivated plasma versus quarantine fresh frozen plasma in thrombotic thrombocytopenic purpura: a multicentric, prospective cohort study. Br J Haematol 2008;143:39–45.

12. Scully M, Longair I, Flynn M, et al. Cryosupernatant and solvent detergent fresh-frozen plasma (Octaplas) usage at a single centre in acute thrombotic thrombocytopenic purpura. Vox Sang 2007;93:154–8.

13. Zeigler ZR, Shadduck RK, Gryn JF, et al, the North American TTP Group. Cryoprecipitate poor plasma does not improve early response in primary adult thrombotic thrombocytopenic purpura (TTP). J Clin Apher 2001;16:19–22.

14. George JN. How I treat patients with thrombotic thrombocytopenic purpura: 2010. Blood 2010;116:4060–9.

15. Lim W, Vesely SK, George JN. The role of rituximab in the management of patients with acquired thrombotic thrombocytopenic purpura. Blood 2015;125: 1526–31.

16. Rock G, Shumak KH, Sutton DM, et al, the Canadian Apheresis Study Group. Cryosupernatant as replacement fluid for plasma exchange in thrombotic thrombocytopenic purpura. Br J Haematol 1996;94:383–6.

17. Scully M, Hunt BJ, Benjamin S, et al. Guidelines on the diagnosis and management of thrombotic thrombocytopenic purpura and other thrombotic microangiopathies. Br J Haematol 2012;158:323–35.

18. Hart D, Sayer R, Miller R, et al. Human immunodeficiency virus associated thrombotic thrombocytopenic purpura—favorable outcome with plasma exchange and prompt initiation of highly active antiretroviral therapy. Br J Haematol 2011;153: 515–9.

19. Rosove MH. Thrombotic microangiopathies. Semin Arthritis Rheum 2014;43: 797–805.

20. Colic E, Dieperink H, Titlestad K, et al. Management of an acute outbreak of diarrhea-associated haemolytic uraemic syndrome with early plasma exchange in adults from southern Denmark: an observational study. Lancet 2011;378: 1089–93.

21. Kielstein JT, Beutel G, Fleig S, et al. Best supportive care and therapeutic plasma exchange with or without eculizumab in Shiga-toxin-producing E. coli O104:H4 induced haemolytic-uraemic syndrome: an analysis of the German STEC-HUS registry. Nephrol Dial Transplant 2012;27:3807–15.

22. Menne J, Nitschke M, Stingele R, et al. Validation of treatment strategies for enterohaemorrhagic Escherichia coli O104:H4 induced haemolytic-uraemic syndrome: case-control study. BMJ 2012;345:e4565.

23. Scheiring J, Andreoli SP, Zimmerheld LB. Treatment and outcome of Shiga-toxin-associated hemolytic uremic syndrome (HUS). Pediatr Nephrol 2008;23: 1749–60.

24. Spinale JM, Ruebner RL, Kaplan BS, et al. Update on Streptococcus pneumonia associated hemolytic uremic syndrome. Curr Opin Pediatr 2013;25:203–8.

25. Loirat C, Saland J, Bitzan M. Management of hemolytic uremic syndrome. Presse Med 2012;41:e115–35.

26. Waters AM, Kerecuk L, Luk D, et al. Hemolytic uremic syndrome associated with invasive pneumococcal disease: the United Kingdom experience. J Pediatr 2007; 151:140–4.

27. Davin JC, van de Kar NC. Advances and challenges in the management of complement-mediated thrombotic microangiopathies. Ther Adv Hematol 2015; 6:171–85.

28. Cataland SR, Wu HM. How I treat: the clinical differentiation and initial treatment of adult patients with atypical hemolytic uremic syndrome. Blood 2014;123: 2478–84.

29. Kennedy GA, Kearey N, Bleakley S, et al. Transplantation-associated thrombotic microangiopathy: effect of concomitant GVHD on efficacy of therapeutic plasma exchange. Bone Marrow Transplant 2010;45:699–704.

30. Choi CM, Schmaier AH, Snell MR, et al. Thrombotic microangiopathy in haematopoietic stem cell transplantation diagnosis and treatment. Drugs 2009;69: 183–98.

31. Ruutu T, Barosi G, Benjamin RJ, et al. Diagnostic criteria for hematopoietic stem cell transplant-associated microangiopathy: results of a consensus process by an International Working Group. Haematologica 2007;92:95–100.

32. Ho VT, Cutler C, Carter S, et al. Blood and marrow transplant clinical trials network toxicity committee consensus summary: thrombotic microangiopathy after hematopoietic stem cell transplantation. Biol Blood Marrow Transplant 2005;11: 571–5.

33. Laskin BL, Goebel J, Davies SM, et al. Small vessel, big trouble in the kidneys and beyond: hematopoietic stem cell transplantation-associated thrombotic microangiopathy. Blood 2011;118:1452–62.

34. Schwimmer J, Nasasdy TA, Spitalnik PF, et al. De novo thrombotic microangiopathy in renal transplant recipients: a comparison of hemolytic uremic syndrome with localized renal thrombotic microangiopathy. Am J Kidney Dis 2003;41:471–9.

35. Reynolds JC, Agodoa LY, Yuan CM, et al. Thrombotic microangiopathy after renal transplantation in the United States. Am J Kidney Dis 2003;42:1058–68.

36. Caires RA, Marques IDB, Repizo LP, et al. De novo thrombotic microangiopathy after kidney transplantation: clinical features, treatment, and long-term patient and graft survival. Transplant Proc 2012;44:2388–90.

37. Elliott MA, Letendre L, Gastineau DA, et al. Cancer-associated microangiopathic hemolytic anemia with thrombocytopenia: an important diagnostic consideration. Eur J Haematol 2010;85:43–50.

38. Houston SA, Hegele RG, Sugar L, et al. Is thrombotic microangiopathy a paraneoplastic phenomenon? Case report and review of the literature. NDT Plus 2014;4:292–4.

39. Oberic L, Buffet M, Schwarzinger M, et al. Cancer awareness in atypical thrombotic microangiopathies. Oncologist 2009;14:769–79.

40. Ducos G, Mariotte E, Galicier L, et al. Metastatic cancer-related thrombotic microangiopathies: a cohort study. Future Oncol 2014;10:1727–34.

41. Favre GA, Touzot M, Fremeaux-Bacchi V, et al. Malignancy and thrombotic micro-angiopathy or atypical haemolytic and uraemic syndrome? Br J Haematol 2014; 166:792–805.

42. Lechner K, Obermeier HL. Cancer-related microangiopathic hemolytic anemia clinical and laboratory features in 168 reported cases. Medicine 2012;91: 195–205.

43. Al-Nouri ZL, Reese JA, Terrell DR, et al. Drug-induced thrombotic microangiop-athy: a systemic review of published reports. Blood 2015;125:616–8.

44. Reese JA, Bougie DW, Curtis BR, et al. Drug-induced thrombotic microangiop-athy: experience of the Oklahoma Registry and the BloodCenter of Wisconsin. Am J Hematol 2015;90:406–10.

45. Kreuter J, Winters JL. Drug-associated thrombotic microangiopathies. Semin Thromb Hemost 2012;38:839–44.

Transfusion Considerations in Pediatric Hematology and Oncology Patients

Rachel S. Bercovitz, MD, MS[a,b],*, Cassandra D. Josephson, MD[c]

KEYWORDS

- Pediatrics • Transfusions • Thrombocytopenia • Anemia
- Red blood cell transfusion • Platelet transfusion • Granulocyte transfusion

KEY POINTS

- Pediatric patients with hypoproliferative cytopenias have unique transfusion requirements when compared with their adult counterparts, and there have been few randomized, controlled trials performed to understand optimal transfusion practices.
- Many pediatric oncologists, hematologists, and transplant physicians report transfusing stable patients to maintain a hemoglobin greater than 7 to 8 g/dL and a platelet count greater than 10 to 20,000 platelets/μL.
- Compared with adult patients, young children have a higher incidence of bleeding with a platelet transfusion threshold of 10,000/μL and maintaining a high hemoglobin in the after-transplant period has deleterious effects in children not seen in adults.
- There are no high-quality data to confirm or refute the benefit of granulocyte transfusions over standard antimicrobial therapy in the prevention or treatment of infections in patients with neutropenia.
- This review compiles data from myriad studies performed in pediatric patients to give readers the knowledge needed to make an informed choice when considering different transfusion management strategies in this patient population.

Neither Dr R.S. Bercovitz nor Dr C.D. Josephson has any commercial or financial conflicts of interest to report.

[a] Medical Sciences Institute, BloodCenter of Wisconsin, 638 North 18th Street, Milwaukee, WI 53233, USA; [b] Department of Pathology and Pediatrics, Medical College of Wisconsin, 8701 W Watertown Plank Rd, Milwaukee, WI 53226, USA; [c] Department of Pathology and Pediatrics, Emory University School of Medicine, Children's Healthcare of Atlanta, 1405 Clifton Road Northeast, Atlanta, GA 30322, USA
* Corresponding author.
E-mail address: rachel.bercovitz@bcw.edu

Hematol Oncol Clin N Am 30 (2016) 695–709
http://dx.doi.org/10.1016/j.hoc.2016.01.010
0889-8588/16/$ – see front matter © 2016 Elsevier Inc. All rights reserved.

hemonc.theclinics.com

INTRODUCTION

Pediatric patients with malignancies or benign hematologic diseases are a heterogeneous group with complicated underlying pathophysiologies leading to their requirements for transfusion therapy. Their ages range from preterm and term neonates, infants, young children, and adolescents, and each of these age groups has unique transfusion requirements. The focus of this review is on transfusion therapies in pediatric patients with hypoproliferative cytopenias, particularly secondary to chemotherapy, hematopoietic stem cell transplant (HSCT), congenital cytopenias, and aplastic anemia (**Table 1**).

EPIDEMIOLOGY OF TRANSFUSIONS IN PEDIATRIC PATIENTS

Overall, pediatric patients are the recipients of 1.1% of plasma, 2.1% of red blood cells (RBC), and 4.8% of platelet transfusions in the United States, which translates to 425,000 units transfused to children in 2011.[1] In adult patients, RBCs and plasma (thawed, fresh frozen [FFP], or plasma frozen) are the 2 most commonly transfused components followed by platelets, cryoprecipitate, and granulocytes.[1] RBCs and platelets are the most commonly transfused components in pediatric patients.[2] Slonim and colleagues[2] published a study using the Pediatric Health Information System data set for transfusion information for more than 1,000,000 pediatric hospital discharges that occurred between 1997 and 2004. This study found approximately 5% of all patients received one or more transfusions during their hospitalization. Neonates (<30 days of age) received 17.5% of the transfusions.[2] According to a single-center retrospective review at an academic tertiary care pediatric hospital, the most commonly transfused patients are those undergoing cardiac surgery (22% of the cohort), premature neonates (21.6%), patients with malignancies (10.9%), and patients with benign hematologic disorders (9.6%).[3]

The complication rate in pediatric patients is approximately 6.2 to 10.7 per 1000 units transfused.[2,4] At a single institution, the rate of complications in pediatric patients was 2.6 times higher than that in adult patients.[4] Pediatric patients were more likely to develop allergic reactions (2.7/1000 vs 1.1/1000 transfusions), febrile nonhemolytic reactions (1.9/1000 vs 0.47/1000 transfusions), and hypotensive reactions (0.29/1000 vs 0.078/1000 transfusions).[4,5] Hemovigilance data should be interpreted with caution because of differences in reporting frequency, but it is important to consider the developmental and underlying disease differences between pediatric and adult transfusion recipients.

RED BLOOD CELL TRANSFUSIONS

RBC transfusions are an integral part of the supportive care for patients with anemia due to bone marrow suppression or failure; however, there have been few randomized, controlled trials (RCTs) designed to investigate optimal RBC transfusion strategies. The only randomized, controlled RBC transfusion trials performed in pediatric patients have evaluated the difference in transfusions and outcomes in neonates[6–8] and critically ill children.[9] In critically ill children, a restrictive transfusion strategy (hemoglobin ≤7 g/dL) resulted in fewer patients receiving transfusions than a liberal strategy (≤9.5 g/dL; 46% vs 98%, P<.001); however, among those children transfused, there was no difference in the number of units transfused (1.9 ± 3.4 vs 1.7 ± 2.1 units per patient, P = .24).[9] There was no difference in morbidity in the 2 cohorts.

In contrast, a retrospective study of pediatric HSCT patients at a single institution demonstrated that a lower threshold of a hemoglobin of 7 g/dL did not decrease

Table 1
Brief summary of transfusion guidelines for pediatric patients with bone marrow suppression

Component	Recommended Dose[35]	Anticipated Result	Indications	Relevant Studies (Reference Number)
Packed RBCs	10–15 mL/kg or 1 unit for patients >25 kg	Hemoglobin increase of 1–2 g/dL	Hemoglobin <7–8 g/dL in stable, uncomplicated patients	9,10,16,26,36
Platelets	10–15 mL/kg (SDP) 1 unit/10 kg body weight (WBD)	20,000–40,000 platelets/μL	Platelet count: <10–20,000/μL: stable, uncomplicated patients <50,000/μL: patients with sickle cell disease undergoing HSCT	19,20,38,39,42
Plasma	10–15 mL/kg	15%–20% increase in factor levels	Coagulopathy associated with multiple factor deficiency	51,53,54
Cryoprecipitate	1–2 units per 10 kg body weight	Fibrinogen increase of 60–100 mg/dL	Fibrinogen level <100 mg/dL	—
Granulocytes	>1 × 10^10 cells/kg	N/A	ANC <500/μL likely to persist ≥5 d AND Bacterial or fungal infection that has not responded to appropriate antimicrobials	67,74,75

Abbreviations: SDP, single-donor apheresis platelet unit; WBD, whole blood-derived platelet unit.
Data from Refs.9,10,16,19,20,26,35,36,38,39,42,51,53,54,67,74,75

the number of transfused patients compared with the cohort of patients with a threshold of 9 g/dL (96% vs 98.5%, respectively; $P = .38$).[10] Patients with the lower transfusion threshold received fewer transfusions (median = 3, interquartile range [2–5] vs 4 [3–8], $P = .002$), which was associated with approximately $1,400 saving in transfusion-related charges.[10] There was no difference in time to engraftment, length of hospital stay, or 100-day mortality, although it is unclear whether this study was sufficiently powered for these outcomes.

A recent *Cochrane Database Review* summarized 19 RCTs that compared restrictive and liberal transfusion strategies in myriad patient populations; only one included adults undergoing HSCT or leukemia therapy.[11,12] This pilot study of 60 adults was designed to investigate whether a liberal transfusion threshold of 12 g/dL of hemoglobin would result in decreased bleeding compared with a restrictive transfusion threshold of 8 g/dL.[12] This pilot study was not powered to evaluate outcomes such as number of RBC transfusions or bleeding incidence, but showed that such a trial would be feasible and safe to perform as a large, multi-institutional RCT.

Based on this pilot study and previous studies in children with leukemia and murine models, which showed high hemoglobin levels were associated with faster neutrophil recovery,[13–15] a trial comparing a hemoglobin threshold of 7 versus 12 g/dL was designed for pediatric patients undergoing HSCT.[16] However, this trial was stopped after enrolling only 6 patients (3 per arm) when all 3 patients in the 12-g/dL arm developed severe veno-occlusive disease (VOD).[16] Not only was the incidence significantly higher in the experimental arm than in the control arm but also the severity of the VOD was higher than historic controls.[16] It is possible that the increased blood viscosity could have decreased sinusoidal blood flow, increasing risk of VOD. Also, the patients in the experimental arm received dramatically more RBC transfusions (3, 9, and 14 vs 2, 1, and 1) than patients in the control arm.[16] Therefore, it is also possible that the RBC transfusions directly contributed to VOD development through the introduction of inflammatory cytokines and RBC microvesicles.[17]

The investigators of this RCT recommend continuing to use the lower transfusion threshold of 7 g/dL,[16] which agrees with what many pediatric oncologists and HSCT physicians report doing.[18,19] In a 2005 survey of members of the American Society for Pediatric Hematology/Oncology (ASPHO) who reside in the United States, Wong and associates[19] found that 56% of pediatric oncologists used a threshold of 7 g/dL or less and 42% used 8 g/dL or less. A survey of HSCT directors at institutions in the Children's Oncology Group revealed that 25% report using a threshold of 7 g/dL or less and 60% use 8 g/dL or less.[18] These responses suggest consistency among practitioners in uncomplicated patients; however, practice varies widely in different clinical situations. For example, in a child with neutropenic fever and tachypnea, approximately 5% of respondents would automatically transfuse at a hemoglobin 7 g/dL or less, 34% would use a threshold of 8 g/dL, 20% would transfuse at a hemoglobin 9 g/dL or less, and 42% would transfuse even if the hemoglobin was greater than 9 g/dL.[19] Among hematologists managing patients with aplastic anemia, 50% report transfusing to maintain a hemoglobin greater than 6 to 8 g/dL and 31% only transfuse symptomatic patients.[20]

Patients undergoing radiation therapy represent a unique challenge with respect to appropriate hemoglobin threshold during treatment. In fact, 48% of respondents report transfusing patients undergoing radiation therapy to maintain a hemoglobin greater than 9 g/dL.[19] This practice stems from reports that patients with head and neck and gynecologic malignancies with low hemoglobin before and during radiation therapy had decreased survival compared with those without anemia.[21–23] However, subsequent phase III trials that used either erythropoiesis-stimulating agents (ESAs) or RBC transfusions to correct anemia in patients undergoing radiation therapy showed that low hemoglobin was associated with decreased survival; however, anemic patients who received ESAs or transfusions actually fared worse than patients in the control arm.[24,25] It is likely that the degree of anemia in these patients is associated with disease severity and therefore portends a poor prognosis and that correction of the anemia fails to mitigate the risk of relapse or progression. There has been one retrospective study published in pediatric patients with central nervous system (CNS) tumors that found hemoglobin less than 10 g/dL during radiation therapy was not associated with local recurrence and overall survival.[26]

Another treatment-related morbidity associated with RBC transfusions is iron overload. Liver iron levels as measured by MRI and serum ferritin are directly correlated with volume of RBCs received during treatment.[27–29] Therefore, patients who have received the most intense therapy for the longest duration are at the highest risk of iron overload.[28,29] This finding is particularly true in patients with high-risk or relapsed cancer who undergo chemotherapy before HSCT.[30,31] Bae and associates[30] found that in children undergoing tandem autologous HSCTs for neuroblastoma, a dose of CD34+ cells was inversely correlated with both volume of RBCs transfused in the aftertransplant period as well as serum ferritin levels. Because of confounders such as disease severity and treatment length and intensity, it can be difficult to isolate the role that iron overload plays in treatment-related morbidity and mortality.[31]

For many patients, once treatment is complete or engraftment after HSCT occurs, RBC transfusions are no longer needed so the expectation is that as these children grow and develop iron levels will decrease.[29] One study found that the ferritin level of most patients decreased to less than 1000 µg/L within 1 year following their last transfusion; however, in a small minority of patients, elevated serum ferritin persisted more than 3 years after their last transfusion.[29] Another small study found persistently elevated liver iron levels as detected by MRI over a year since the patients' last transfusions.[32]

These myriad studies suggest that a restrictive transfusion strategy, which is commonly used in pediatric hematology, oncology, and HSCT patients not only reduces number of transfusions but also may be associated with decreased morbidity and mortality. Patients undergoing HSCT for sickle cell disease have unique RBC transfusion needs; routine practice includes maintaining hemoglobin S percent less than 30% during the pretransplant preparation phase and to maintain a hemoglobin greater than 9 g/dL aftertransplant until RBC engraftment occurs.[33,34]

In addition to transfusion threshold, dosage of RBCs is another issue. The recommendation for dosing in young children is 10 to 15 mL/kg,[35] but in older children, like adult patients, there is the option for single-unit versus double-unit transfusions. A study of 139 adult oncology patients demonstrated that a single-unit policy reduced RBC transfusions by 25% and did not increase transfusion frequency.[36] Similar studies need to be performed in adolescents.

Although a liberal transfusion strategy may be associated with adverse outcomes in pediatric patients as evidenced by the small study that found transfusing to maintain a hemoglobin greater than 12 g/dL was associated with adverse outcomes in patients undergoing HSCT[16] (realizing that a threshold of 7–8 g/dL is commonly used),[18,19] there are additional factors that should be considered in pediatric patients. The National Heart, Lung, and Blood Institute has recognized that multicenter RCTs are needed to better understand the impact that RBC transfusion threshold has on outcomes such as quality of life, growth and development in young children, incidence of bleeding events, impact on the immune system and incidence of infections, return of hematopoiesis, and event-free and overall survival.[37] These trials can be incorporated into cancer treatment trials to better understand the unique needs of patients receiving different treatment regimens.

PLATELET TRANSFUSIONS

Bleeding is a common complication in patients with hypoproliferative thrombocyto-penia. Given risks for HLA alloimmunization and other adverse effects of platelet trans-fusions, reducing unnecessary transfusions without increasing bleeding risk is a priority. There have been numerous trials to investigate optimal platelet transfusion strategies to minimize bleeding risk. Only one of these trials, the Platelet Dose (PLADO) trial, included pediatric patients, which investigated whether a dose of 1.1×10^{11}, 2.2×10^{11}, and 4.4×10^{11} platelets per square meter per transfusion would have an impact on bleeding incidence.[38,39] This study used a prophylactic transfusion threshold of 10,000 platelets/μL for all patients.[39] Overall, in the 1272 patients who received a platelet transfusion, the incidence of at least one clinically significant bleeding episode was about 70% in all treatment cohorts.[39]

In a subgroup analysis of the 200 patients 18 years of age or younger, pediatric pa-tients were found to have a significantly increased incidence of bleeding compared with adults.[38] Bleeding incidence was inversely correlated with age: 86%, 88%, 77%, and 67%, for ages 0 to 5, 6 to 12, 13 to 18, and 19 years and older, respectively ($P<.001$).[38] In fact, among pediatric patients, those aged 0 to 5 undergoing autologous stem cell transplant had the highest incidence of bleeding (93%). These findings high-light the importance of performing high-quality RCTs in pediatric patients and not merely extrapolating data from adult trials to pediatric patients. Of the 2 studies that investigated a prophylactic transfusion threshold of 10,000/μL compared with a ther-apeutic transfusion-only strategy in patients 16 years old and older, autologous trans-plant patients had a significantly lower incidence of clinically significantly bleeding than patients being treated for a hematologic malignancy (with either chemotherapy or allogeneic HSCT).[40,41] Of note, both of these trials found that patients on a thera-peutic transfusion-only regimen had a higher incidence of bleeding compared with those receiving prophylactic platelet transfusions.[40,41]

Although this study found no difference in bleeding incidence between the different dosage cohorts, subjects who received a higher dose of platelets overall received fewer platelet transfusions: 3.6 platelet transfusions per person in the high-dose group compared with 4.5 and 6.1 transfusions per person in the medium- and low-dose groups, respectively.[39] There was also a longer time between transfusions: median of 2.9 days in the high-dose group compared with 1.9 and 1.1 days in the medium- and low-dose groups, respectively ($P<.001$).[39] Current recommendations for platelet dose are 10 to 15 mL/kg of body weight.[35] The data from the PLADO trial suggest that patients for whom dosing at the higher end of this range may have a longer interval between transfusions and receive fewer transfusions, which reduces donor expo-sures. These data also suggest that there is little benefit to transfusing more than a sin-gle apheresis donor unit as a method of decreasing bleeding risk.

All of the platelet transfusion trials in both pediatric and adult patients have been performed in the inpatient setting. Outpatient management of hypoproliferative throm-bocytopenia is not well-studied, although most providers use a threshold of 10,000 or 20,000/μL.[18–20] In a survey of pediatric oncologists, 54% of respondents reported using a prophylactic transfusion threshold of 10,000/μL and 42% reported using 20,000/μL.[19] Similarly, 44% of pediatric HSCT directors reported using a prophylactic threshold of 10,000/μL and 47% use 20,000/μL.[18] In a survey of 18 children's hospitals who care for patients with aplastic anemia, 91% of respondents reported using a pro-phylactic platelet transfusion threshold of 10,000/μL, whereas 64% use 20,000/μL as the threshold in patients receiving antithymocyte globulin and 28% use a threshold between 30 and 50,000/μL.[20] In general, a platelet transfusion threshold of 10,000 to 20,000/µL in stable patients with hypoproliferative thrombocytopenia minimizes both bleeding risk and exposure to platelet transfusions. One notable exception to this group is children and young adults undergoing HSCT for sickle cell disease, who have an increased risk of neurologic complications in the after-transplant period.[42] In a case series of 28 pediatric patients, 3 patients developed intracranial hemorrhage, and in 2 cases, this bleeding was fatal.[42] All 3 of these patients had a history of stroke before transplant, indicating this is a particularly high-risk group. In the after-transplant time period, platelet count should be maintained greater than 50,000/µL in order to minimize risk of hemorrhagic stroke.[33,34,43]

Although there appears to be consensus for management of stable thrombocytopenic patients, there are significant variability and little data regarding transfusion practices for patients undergoing a procedure such as bone marrow biopsy or lumbar puncture. Of the respondents from the ASPHO survey, for patients undergoing a lumbar puncture, 8% would use a threshold of less than 10,000/µL, 26% would use a threshold less than 20,000/µL, 48% would transfuse if the platelet count were between 25 and 50,000/µL, and 19% would transfuse if platelets were less than 50,000/µL.[19] The rate of severe complications (eg, spinal subdural hematoma or spontaneous hemorrhage) in children undergoing lumbar puncture is quite low, even at platelet counts of less than 20,000/µL.[44] However, traumatic lumbar puncture occurs at a rate of 10% to 29%,[45–49] and in patients with circulating peripheral blasts, this can adversely affect progression-free survival and increase risk of CNS relapse.[47–49]

There are many variables that can have an impact on risk of traumatic lumbar puncture, including patient age, race, and body mass index; provider experience; and time since previous lumbar puncture.[46,47] Platelet count is inversely correlated with the risk of traumatic lumbar puncture.[46,47] In multivariable regression models, platelet counts 0 to 25,000/µL, 26,000 to 50,000/µL, 51,000 to 75,000/µL, and 76,000 to 100,000 had an odds ratio (OR) of 1.8, 1.4, 1.5, and 1.4 compared with platelet counts greater than 100,000/µL were associated with increased risk of traumatic and blood lumbar punctures.[46] Shaikh and colleagues[47] found a similar risk in patients with a platelet count less than 100,000/µL. An important note of these studies is that, in general, there was no difference in risk of traumatic lumbar puncture, if the platelet count was between 20,000 and 30,000/µL and 100,000 µL.[44,46,50]

Although there are associations between platelet count less than 100,000/µL and risk of traumatic lumbar puncture and between traumatic lumbar puncture with circulating blasts and risk of CNS relapse, there have been no studies performed that have found a direct link between platelet count at the time of initial lumbar puncture and event-free survival. In newly diagnosed patients with leukemia who often present profoundly thrombocytopenic, it may be difficult to increase their platelet count greater than 100,000/µL, and doing so may cause fluid overload and delay diagnosis and treatment initiation. Therefore, the decision to transfuse a patient before lumbar puncture to achieve a specific platelet count should be made on an individual basis that considers the other risk factors associated with traumatic or bloody lumbar puncture and the patient's underlying disease.

PLASMA TRANSFUSIONS

Plasma transfusions are not routinely given to pediatric hematology, oncology, and HSCT patients; the bone marrow suppression that leads to RBC and platelet transfusion requirements does not affect coagulation factors. In a study of pediatric tertiary care hospitals, only 7% of patients who received plasma transfusions were on the Hematology or Oncology services.[51] The most common indication for plasma transfusion in pediatric oncology patients is treatment of the coagulopathy associated with newly diagnosed promyelocytic leukemia.[52]

There have been 2 RCTs that have investigated the use of FFP to prevent VOD in the after-HSCT period.[53,54] The proposed mechanism by which plasma transfusions could prevent VOD would be replacement of ADAMTS13, which Park and colleagues[55] found was decreased in children who developed VOD compared with those who did not. This group performed a small RCT (47 patients: 15 children and 32 adults).[53] Subjects were randomized to receive FFP twice weekly during conditioning and for the first 28 days after HSCT.[53] In this study, FFP was specifically dosed to maintain a plasma ADAMTS13 level 30% of normal.[53] None of the pediatric patients in this trial developed VOD, but of the group that did not receive FFP, 3 of 20 developed VOD, and no patients in the FFP cohort developed VOD (OR 0.12, 95% confidence interval [CI]: 0.01–2.56).[53] A second, larger RCT included both pediatric (children >5 years old) and adults, but did not include a separate pediatric analysis. Three hundred thirty-six patients were randomized to receive either 2 units of FFP and heparin or heparin alone during conditioning.[54] FFP administration did not reduce VOD incidence (OR 1.27, 95% CI: 0.28–5.60).[54] A recent *Cochrane Database Review* found that combined, the OR of developing VOD in patients receiving prophylactic FFP transfusions was 0.66 with a 95% CI of 0.20 to 2.17.[56] There is no evidence to support prophylactic FFP transfusions for the prevention of VOD in HSCT patients at this time.

GRANULOCYTE TRANSFUSIONS

Prolonged neutropenia increases a patient's risk of developing life-threatening bacterial and fungal infections, which are major causes of morbidity and mortality in children undergoing chemotherapy or HSCT. The data have been mixed with regards to the efficacy of granulocyte transfusions in the prevention and treatment of infections in the setting of neutropenia or neutrophil dysfunction.[57,58] There are no clear guidelines for the clinical indications, but the general consensus is that patients for whom granulocytes may be appropriate include those with (1) absolute neutrophil count (ANC) less than 500 neutrophils/μL or known neutrophil dysfunction (such as in patients with chronic granulomatous disease) and (2) clinical evidence of bacterial or fungal infection that has (3) not responded to appropriate antimicrobial therapy.[58] Other considerations include expected timing of recovery of hematopoiesis; patients whose marrow function is expected to imminently recover may derive less benefit from granulocyte transfusions than individuals for whom neutrophil recovery is unlikely in the following 5 to 10 days.[58,59]

Adverse events occur in approximately 15% to 20% of granulocyte transfusions.[60–62] The most common side effects of granulocyte transfusions are fever and hypotension. However, among patients with underlying pulmonary disease, either related or unrelated to the present infection, there is an increased risk of respiratory deterioration during or shortly after granulocyte transfusion.[58,60,62,63] There have been reports of liposomal amphotericin B administration within 4 hours following granulocyte transfusions, which increases risk of respiratory failure.[64] However, subsequent studies have not substantiated these findings and have suggested that it is more likely that the underlying pneumonia caused by either *Candida* sp or *Aspergillus* sp is more likely to predispose patients to pulmonary complications rather than the Amphotericin B.[65]

There are limited data with respect to the efficacy of granulocyte transfusions in children with neutropenia or neutrophil recovery because few modern RCTs have included pediatric patients. In a 2005 *Cochrane Database Review* of the efficacy of granulocyte transfusions in treating infections in patients with neutropenia or neutrophil dysfunction (updated in 2010),[66] the only RCTs that included children were published in 1977 and 1982.[67–70] In these 4 studies, a total of 93 patients received granulocyte transfusions in addition to antimicrobial therapy and 93 patients received only antimicrobials, and approximately 50% of all subjects were in the trial performed by Winston and colleagues.[67–70] In all trials, pediatric patients made up a small subset of enrolled subjects (<35%) and only Alavi and associates[67] included pediatric-specific outcome data.

Two of the smaller trials found a benefit to granulocyte transfusions with respect to infection-related mortality[68,69]; however, the larger trial by Winston and associates[70] demonstrated no survival benefit attributable to the receipt of granulocyte transfusions. Granulocyte transfusions may have conferred a survival benefit to the subset of patients who had persistent neutropenia secondary to delayed hematopoietic recovery.[67,70] Among the pediatric patients in the study performed by Alavi and colleagues,[67] 3 of 4 patients (75%) in the control group survived (aged 8–18) and 5 of 6 (83%) patients in the granulocyte transfusion cohort survived (aged 9–18). The investigators did not provide a separate statistical analysis for the pediatric subjects.

Since that *Cochrane Review* was published, there have been several single-arm retrospective studies in pediatric patients with neutropenia. These case series showed that a relatively high percentage (approximately 90%) of pediatric patients treated with granulocytes for acute infection were able to clear their infection, with 72% to 89.5% of patients surviving at least 1 month following treatment.[63,71–74] Complication rates varied between 0% and 46%, but all investigators concluded granulocyte transfusions were sufficiently safe to consider their use.[63,71–74]

Most of the granulocyte transfusion trials have only included patients with neutropenia secondary to chemotherapy or HSCT; however, Wang and colleagues[61] recently published a case series of 56 patients with severe aplastic anemia (SAA) and severe bacterial and fungal infections who were treated with granulocyte transfusions in combination with granulocyte-colony stimulating factor (GCSF). Patients aged 6 to 65 years old were included in this study and had received immunosuppressive therapy for their SAA, which included antilymphocyte globulin or antithymocyte globulin in combination with cyclosporine. Nine patients had been treated with cyclosporine and androgen therapy. Overall 30-day survival was 89%, and 13.8% of granulocyte transfusions were associated with adverse events (most commonly fever and chills, allergy, and dyspnea).[61] These outcomes appear to be on par with other retrospective case series,[63,71–74] suggesting that granulocyte transfusions are equally effective in this patient population.

Because the studies performed in the 1970s and 1980s were inconsistent in their findings, a phase III RCT comparing granulocyte transfusions to standard antimicrobial therapy in 74 patients with chemotherapy-induced hypoproliferative neutropenia was performed.[59] There were no pediatric subjects in the granulocyte transfusion arm, although in the control arm, the youngest subject was 14 years old. This trial failed to demonstrate the benefit of granulocyte transfusions in improving 28- and 100-day mortality.[59] Some weaknesses of this trial included that neutrophil recovery occurred more quickly than anticipated in the control arm; there were delays in granulocyte collection and administration, and despite administrated of GCSF to donors, the dose of granulocytes administered to patients was relatively low.[59]

The RING (*Resolving Infection in Neutropenia with Granulocytes*) trial sought to address the question of whether efficacy of granulocyte transfusions was uncertain due to inadequate dosing in prior trials. Subjects with neutropenia due to HSCT or treatment with chemotherapy were randomized to receive standard antimicrobial therapy with or without granulocyte transfusions.[75] Granulocytes were collected from donors who had received GCSF (480 μg) and oral dexamethasone (8 mg) 12 hours before collection in an effort to increase granulocyte yield. The study initially anticipated enrolling 236 subjects, but because of slow enrollment, closed in 2013 after enrolling only 114 subjects (58 in the control arm, 56 in the granulocyte transfusion arm).[75] Of these 114 subjects, only 10 were children less than 18 years old. Only preliminary results are available; however, there was no difference in the patients who were alive and demonstrated a microbial response at 42 days following enrollment between the control and granulocyte transfusion arms (42.9% and 41.7%, respectively).[75]

In addition to treating severe infection, granulocytes have been administered to patients to prevent infections during the period of neutropenia following intensive chemotherapy or HSCT.[57] A recent *Cochrane Database Review* included 11 RCTs comparing prophylactic granulocyte transfusions versus standard of care. Nine of these studies were published before 1985, and the remaining 2 by Oza and associates[76] and Vij and associates[77] were only quasi-randomized.[57] In both of these studies, granulocytes were donated by the HLA-matched sibling donor, who provided the stem cells, and assignment to the granulocyte-transfusion arm was based on donor-recipient ABO compatibility.[76,77] In the 9 studies wherein infection incidence was an outcome of interest, the incidence of bacteremia or fungemia is reduced in recipients of prophylactic granulocyte transfusions (risk ratio: 0.45, 95% CI: 0.30–0.65); this reduction is more pronounced in the trials that administered a higher dose of granulocytes.[57] There was no difference in all-cause 30-day mortality (0.92, 0.63–1.36) or 30-day infection-related mortality (0.69, 0.33–1.44).[57] Although some of the studies included in this review enrolled pediatric subjects, none provided a separate analysis of outcomes in children.

Given the advancements in antimicrobial therapy and infection prevention in neutropenic patients that have occurred in the last 30 years, it is uncertain whether this magnitude of benefit in the prevention of infection would be seen today. In summary, despite recent attempts at performing large RCTs to definitively answer the question of benefit of granulocyte transfusions that was raised by these early trials and retrospective reviews, there are still no high-quality data to confirm or refute the benefit of granulocyte transfusions over standard antimicrobial therapy in the prevention or treatment of infections in patients with neutropenia.

REFERENCES

1. Report of the US Department of Health and Human Services. The 2011 National Blood Collection and Utilization Survey Report. Washington, DC: US Department of Health and Human Services, Office of the Assistant Secretary for Health; 2013.
2. Slonim AD, Joseph JG, Turenne WM, et al. Blood transfusions in children: a multi-institutional analysis of practices and complications. Transfusion 2008;48(1): 73–80.
3. Gauvin F, Champagne MA, Robillard P, et al. Long-term survival rate of pediatric patients after blood transfusion. Transfusion 2008;48(5):801–8.
4. Oakley FD, Woods M, Arnold S, et al. Transfusion reactions in pediatric compared with adult patients: a look at rate, reaction type, and associated products. Transfusion 2015;55(3):563–70.
5. Savage WJ. The unique challenges of hemovigilance for pediatric patients. Transfusion 2015;55(3):466–7.

6. Bell EF, Strauss RG, Widness JA, et al. Randomized trial of liberal versus restrictive guidelines for red blood cell transfusion in preterm infants. Pediatrics 2005; 115(6):1685–91.

7. Kirpalani H, Whyte RK, Andersen C, et al. The Premature Infants in Need of Transfusion (PINT) study: a randomized, controlled trial of a restrictive (low) versus liberal (high) transfusion threshold for extremely low birth weight infants. J Pediatr 2006;149(3):301–7.

8. Whyte RK, Kirpalani H, Asztalos EV, et al. Neurodevelopmental outcome of extremely low birth weight infants randomly assigned to restrictive or liberal hemoglobin thresholds for blood transfusion. Pediatrics 2009;123(1):207–13.

9. Lacroix J, Hebert PC, Hutchison JS, et al. Transfusion strategies for patients in pediatric intensive care units. N Engl J Med 2007;356(16):1609–19.

10. Lightdale JR, Randolph AG, Tran CM, et al. Impact of a conservative red blood cell transfusion strategy in children undergoing hematopoietic stem cell transplantation. Biol Blood Marrow Transplant 2012;18(5):813–7.

11. Carson JL, Carless PA, Hebert PC. Transfusion thresholds and other strategies for guiding allogeneic red blood cell transfusion. Cochrane Database Syst Rev 2012;(4):CD002042.

12. Webert KE, Cook RJ, Couban S, et al. A multicenter pilot-randomized controlled trial of the feasibility of an augmented red blood cell transfusion strategy for patients treated with induction chemotherapy for acute leukemia or stem cell transplantation. Transfusion 2008;48(1):81–91.

13. Smith PJ, Jackson CW, Dow LW, et al. Effect of hypertransfusion on bone marrow regeneration in sublethally irradiated mice. I. enhanced granulopoietic recovery. Blood 1980;56(1):52–7.

14. de Montpellier C, Cornu G, Rodhain J, et al. Myeloid stem cell kinetics in children hypertransfused during remission induction of acute lymphoblastic leukemia. Blood Cells 1982;8(2):439–44.

15. Toogood IR, Ekert H, Smith PJ. Controlled study of hypertransfusion during remission induction in childhood acute lymphocytic leukaemia. Lancet 1978;2(8095): 862–4.

16. Robitaille N, Lacroix J, Alexandrov L, et al. Excess of veno-occlusive disease in a randomized clinical trial on a higher trigger for red blood cell transfusion after bone marrow transplantation: a Canadian blood and marrow transplant group trial. Biol Blood Marrow Transplant 2013;19(3):468–73.

17. Sweeney J, Kouttab N, Kurtis J. Stored red blood cell supernatant facilitates thrombin generation. Transfusion 2009;49(8):1569–79.

18. Bercovitz RS, Quinones RR. A survey of transfusion practices in pediatric hematopoietic stem cell transplant patients. J Pediatr Hematol Oncol 2013;35(2): e60–3.

19. Wong EC, Perez-Albuerne E, Moscow JA, et al. Transfusion management strategies: a survey of practicing pediatric hematology/oncology specialists. Pediatr Blood Cancer 2005;44(2):119–27.

20. Williams DA, Bennett C, Bertuch A, et al. Diagnosis and treatment of pediatric acquired aplastic anemia (AAA): an initial survey of the North American Pediatric Aplastic Anemia Consortium (NAPAAC). Pediatr Blood Cancer 2014;61(5): 869–74.

21. Macdonald G, Hurman DC. Influence of anaemia in patients with head and neck cancer receiving adjuvant postoperative radiotherapy in the Grampian region. Clin Oncol (R Coll Radiol) 2004;16(1):63–70.

22. Serkies K, Badzio A, Jassem J. Clinical relevance of hemoglobin level in cervical cancer patients administered definitive radiotherapy. Acta Oncol 2006;45(6): 695–701.

23. Bhide SA, Ahmed M, Rengarajan V, et al. Anemia during sequential induction chemotherapy and chemoradiation for head and neck cancer: the impact of blood transfusion on treatment outcome. Int J Radiat Oncol Biol Phys 2009; 73(2):391–8.

24. Hoff CM, Lassen P, Eriksen JG, et al. Does transfusion improve the outcome for HNSCC patients treated with radiotherapy? Results from the randomized DA-HANCA 5 and 7 trials. Acta Oncol 2011;50(7):1006–14.

25. Lambin P, Ramaekers BL, van Mastrigt GA, et al. Erythropoietin as an adjuvant treatment with (chemo) radiation therapy for head and neck cancer. Cochrane Database Syst Rev 2009;(3):CD006158.

26. Chow E, Danjoux CE, Pataki I, et al. Effect of hemoglobin on radiotherapy response in children with medulloblastoma: should patients with a low hemoglobin be transfused? Med Pediatr Oncol 1999;32:395–7.

27. de Ville de Goyet M, Moniotte S, Robert A, et al. Iron overload in children undergoing cancer treatments. Pediatr Blood Cancer 2013;60(12):1982–7.

28. Amid A, Barrowman N, Vijenthira A, et al. Risk factors for hyperferritinemia secondary to red blood cell transfusions in pediatric cancer patients. Pediatr Blood Cancer 2013;60(10):1671–5.

29. Rascon J, Rageliene L, Stankeviciene S, et al. An assessment of iron overload in children treated for cancer and nonmalignant hematologic disorders. Eur J Pediatr 2014;173(9):1137–46.

30. Bae SJ, Kang C, Sung KW, et al. Iron overload during follow-up after tandem high-dose chemotherapy and autologous stem cell transplantation in patients with high-risk neuroblastoma. J Korean Med Sci 2012;27(4):363–9.

31. Nottage K, Gurney JG, Smeltzer M, et al. Trends in transfusion burden among long-term survivors of childhood hematological malignancies. Leuk Lymphoma 2013;54(8):1719–23.

32. Sait S, Zaghloul N, Patel A, et al. Transfusion related iron overload in pediatric oncology patients treated at a tertiary care centre and treatment with chelation therapy. Pediatr Blood Cancer 2014;61(12):2319–20.

33. Bernaudin F, Socie G, Kuentz M, et al. Long-term results of related myeloablative stem-cell transplantation to cure sickle cell disease. Blood 2007;110(7):2749–56.

34. McPherson ME, Anderson AR, Haight AE, et al. Transfusion management of sickle cell patients during bone marrow transplantation with matched sibling donor. Transfusion 2009;49(9):1977–86.

35. Josephson CD, Sloan SR. Pediatric transfusion medicine. In: Hoffman R, Benz EJ, Silberstein LE, et al, editors. Hematology: basic principles and practice. 6th edition. Philadelphia (PA): Elsevier; 2013. p. 1765–71.

36. Berger MD, Gerber B, Arn K, et al. Significant reduction of red blood cell transfusion requirements by changing from a double-unit to a single-unit transfusion policy in patients receiving intensive chemotherapy or stem cell transplantation. Haematologica 2012;97(1):116–22.

37. Spitalnik SL, Triulzi D, Devine DV, et al. 2015 Proceedings of the National Heart, Lung, and Blood Institute's State of the Science in Transfusion Medicine symposium. Transfusion 2015;55(9):2282–90.

38. Josephson CD, Granger S, Assmann SF, et al. Bleeding risks are higher in children versus adults given prophylactic platelet transfusions for treatment-induced hypoproliferative thrombocytopenia. Blood 2012;120(4):748–60.

39. Slichter SJ, Kaufman RM, Assmann SF, et al. Dose of prophylactic platelet transfusions and prevention of hemorrhage. N Engl J Med 2010;362(7):600–13.

40. Wandt H, Schaefer-Eckart K, Wendelin K, et al. Therapeutic platelet transfusion versus routine prophylactic transfusion in patients with haematological malignancies: an open-label, multicentre, randomised study. Lancet 2012;380(9850): 1309–16.

41. Stanworth SJ, Estcourt LJ, Powter G, et al. A no-prophylaxis platelet-transfusion strategy for hematologic cancers. N Engl J Med 2013;368(19):1771–80.

42. Walters MC, Sullivan KM, Bernaudin F, et al. Neurologic complications after allogeneic marrow transplantation for sickle cell anemia. Blood 1995;85(4):879–84.

43. Walters MC, Patience M, Leisenring W, et al. Stable mixed hematopoietic chimerism after bone marrow transplantation for sickle cell anemia. Biol Blood Marrow Transplant 2001;7(12):665–73.

44. Howard SC, Gajjar A, Ribeiro RC, et al. Safety of lumbar puncture for children with acute lymphoblastic leukemia and thrombocytopenia. JAMA 2000;284(17): 2222–4.

45. Gajjar A, Harrison PL, Sandlund JT, et al. Traumatic lumbar puncture at diagnosis adversely affects outcome in childhood acute lymphoblastic leukemia. Blood 2000;96:3381–4.

46. Howard SC, Gajjar AJ, Cheng C, et al. Risk factors for traumatic and bloody lumbar puncture in children with acute lymphoblastic leukemia. JAMA 2002;288(16): 2001–7.

47. Shaikh F, Voicu L, Tole S, et al. The risk of traumatic lumbar punctures in children with acute lymphoblastic leukaemia. Eur J Cancer 2014;50(8):1482–9.

48. Burger B, Zimmermann M, Mann G, et al. Diagnostic cerebrospinal fluid examination in children with acute lymphoblastic leukemia: significance of low leukocyte counts with blasts or traumatic lumbar puncture. J Clin Oncol 2003;21(2): 184–8.

49. Cancela CS, Murao M, Viana MB, et al. Incidence and risk factors for central nervous system relapse in children and adolescents with acute lymphoblastic leukemia. Rev Bras Hematol Hemoter 2012;34(6):436–41.

50. Ruell J, Karuvattil R, Wynn R, et al. Platelet count has no influence on traumatic and bloody lumbar puncture in children undergoing intrathecal chemotherapy. Br J Haematol 2007;136(2):347–8.

51. Puetz J, Witmer C, Huang YS, et al. Widespread use of fresh frozen plasma in US children's hospitals despite limited evidence demonstrating a beneficial effect. J Pediatr 2012;160(2):210–5.e1.

52. Senz MA, Grimwade D, Tallman MS, et al. Management of acute promyelocytic leukemia: recommendations from an expert panel on behalf of the European LeukemiaNet. Blood 2009;113(9):1875–91.

53. Matsumoto M, Kawa K, Uemura M, et al. Prophylactic fresh frozen plasma may prevent development of hepatic VOD after stem cell transplantation via ADAMTS13-mediated restoration of von Willebrand factor plasma levels. Biol Blood Marrow Transplant 2007;40(3):251–9.

54. Yannaki E, Constantinou V, Baliakas P, et al. Intravenous versus oral busulfan administration results into a dramatic reduction of veno-occlusive disease (VOD) incidence in a randomised trial assessing fresh frozen plasma+heparin versus heparin-alone as anti-VOD prophylaxis. Biol Blood Marrow Transplant 2012;47:S198.

55. Park YD, Yoshioka A, Kawa K, et al. Impaired activity of plasma von Willebrand factor-cleaving protease may predict the occurrence of hepatic veno-occlusive disease after stem cell transplantation. Bone Marrow Transplant 2002;29:789–94.

56. Cheuk DK, Chiang AK, Ha SY, et al. Interventions for prophylaxis of hepatic veno-occlusive disease in people undergoing haematopoietic stem cell transplantation. Cochrane Database Syst Rev 2015;(5):CD009311.

57. Estcourt LJ, Stanworth S, Doree C, et al. Granulocyte transfusions for preventing infections in people with neutropenia or neutrophil dysfunction. Cochrane Database Syst Rev 2015;(6):CD005341.

58. Marfin AA, Price TH. Granulocyte transfusion therapy. J Intensive Care Med 2015; 30(2):79–88.

59. Seidel MG, Peters C, Wacker A, et al. Randomized phase III study of granulocyte transfusions in neutropenic patients. Bone Marrow Transplant 2008;42(10): 679–84.

60. Kim KH, Lim HJ, Kim JS, et al. Therapeutic granulocyte transfusions for the treatment of febrile neutropenia in patients with hematologic diseases: a 10-year experience at a single institute. Cytotherapy 2011;13(4):490–8.

61. Wang H, Wu Y, Fu R, et al. Granulocyte transfusion combined with granulocyte colony stimulating factor in severe infection patients with severe aplastic anemia: a single center experience from China. PLoS One 2014;9(2):e88148.

62. Grigull L, Pulver N, Goudeva L, et al. G-CSF mobilised granulocyte transfusions in 32 paediatric patients with neutropenic sepsis. Support Care Cancer 2006;14(9): 910–6.

63. Diaz R, Soundar E, Hartman SK, et al. Granulocyte transfusions for children with infection and neutropenia or granulocyte dysfunction. Pediatr Hematol Oncol 2014;31(5):425–34.

64. Wright DG, Robichaud KJ, Pizzo PA, et al. Lethal pulmonary reactions associated with the combined use of amphotericin B and leukocyte transfusions. N Engl J Med 1981;304(20):1185–9.

65. Bow EJ, Schroeder ML, Louie TJ. Pulmonary complications in patients receiving granulocyte transfusions and amphotericin B. Can Med Assoc J 1984;130(5): 593–7.

66. Stanworth SJ, Massey E, Hyde C, et al. Granulocyte transfusions for treating infections in patients with neutropenia or neutrophil dysfunction. Cochrane Database Syst Rev 2005;(3):CD005339.

67. Alavi JB, Root RK, Djerassi I, et al. A randomized clinical trial of granulocyte transfusions for infection in acute leukemia. N Engl J Med 1977;296(13):706–11.

68. Herzig RH, Herzig GP, Graw RG Jr, et al. Successful granulocyte transfusion therapy for gram-negative septicemia. A prospectively randomized controlled study. N Engl J Med 1977;296(13):701–5.

69. Vogler WR, Winton EF. A controlled study of the efficacy of granulocyte transfusions in patients with neutropenia. Am J Med 1977;63(4):548–55.

70. Winston DJ, Ho WG, Gale RP. Therapeutic granulocyte transfusions for documented infections. Ann Intern Med 1982;97(4):509–15.

71. Oymak Y, Ayhan Y, Karapinar TH, et al. Granulocyte transfusion experience in pediatric neutropenic fever: split product can be an alternative? Transfus Apher Sci 2015;53(3):348–52.

72. Sachs UJ, Reiter A, Walter T, et al. Safety and efficacy of therapeutic early onset granulocyte transfusions in pediatric patients with neutropenia and severe infections. Transfusion 2006;46(11):1909–14.

73. Atay D, Ozturk G, Akcay A, et al. Effect and safety of granulocyte transfusions in pediatric patients with febrile neutropenia or defective granulocyte functions. J Pediatr Hematol Oncol 2011;33(6):e220–5.
74. Seidel MG, Minkov M, Witt V, et al. Granulocyte transfusions in children and young adults: does the dose matter? J Pediatr Hematol Oncol 2009;31(3): 166–72.
75. Price TH, Boeckh M, Harrison RW, et al. Efficacy of transfusion with granulocytes from G-CSF/dexamethasone-treated donors in neutropenic patients with infection. Blood 2015;126(18):2153–61.
76. Oza A, Hallemeier C, Goodnough L, et al. Granulocyte-colony-stimulating factor-mobilized prophylactic granulocyte transfusions given after allogeneic peripheral blood progenitor cell transplantation result in a modest reduction of febrile days and intravenous antibiotic usage. Transfusion 2006;46(1):14–23.
77. Vij R, DiPersio JF, Venkatraman P, et al. Donor CMV serostatus has no impact on CMV viremia or disease when prophylactic granulocyte transfusions are given following allogeneic peripheral blood stem cell transplantation. Blood 2003; 101(5):2067–9.

Index

Hematol Oncol Clin N Am 30 (2016) 711–721
http://dx.doi.org/10.1016/S0889-8588(16)30046-6
0889-8588/16/$ – see front matter © 2016 Elsevier Inc. All rights reserved.

Printed and bound by CPI Group (UK) Ltd, Croydon, CR0 4YY

03/10/2024

01040388-0019